IRRITABLE BOWEL SYNDROME

DIAGNOSIS, PATHOGENESIS AND TREATMENT OPTIONS

DIGESTIVE DISEASES - RESEARCH AND CLINICAL DEVELOPMENTS

DIGESTIVE DISEASES - RESEARCH AND CLINICAL DEVELOPMENTS

IRRITABLE BOWEL SYNDROME

DIAGNOSIS, PATHOGENESIS AND TREATMENT OPTIONS

MAGDY EL-SALHY

D. GUNDERSEN

J. G. HATLEBAKK

AND

T. HAUSKEN

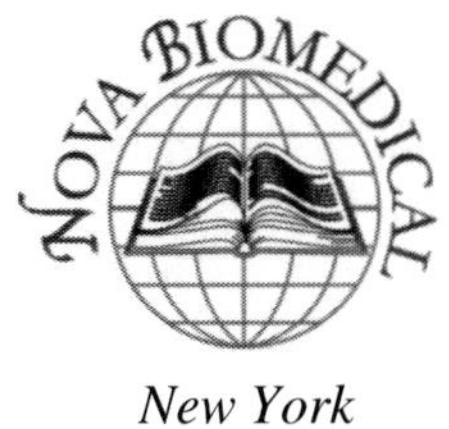

NOVA BIOMEDICAL

New York

For permission to use material from this book please contact us:
Telephone 631-231-7269; Fax 631-231-8175
Web Site: http://www.novapublishers.com

NOTICE TO THE READER

Library of Congress Cataloging-in-Publication Data

Library of Congress Control Number: 2012936702

ISBN: 978-1-63321-244-2

Published by Nova Science Publishers, Inc. ✝ New York

*To the maestro,
the artist,
the administrator
and the student,
and to all those they represent*

Contents

About the Authors

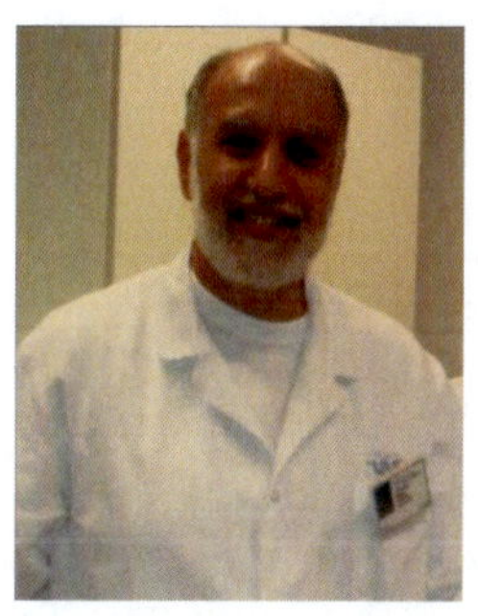

Magdy El-Salhy is Professor of Gastroenterology and Hepatology, School of Medicine, University of Bergen and consultant gastroenterologist at Stord Hospital, Norway. He completed his PhD (Medicine) in 1981 and his MD in 1989, both at Uppsala University, Sweden. He has published 142 papers: 121 original articles and 21 invited reviews and book chapters. He is on the editorial board of seven international journals and associated editor-in-chief of "World Journal of Gastroenterology". His research field for the last 40 years has been the neuroendocrine system of the gut, from basic science to clinical applications. During the last 10 years he has been engaged with research on irritable bowel syndrome.

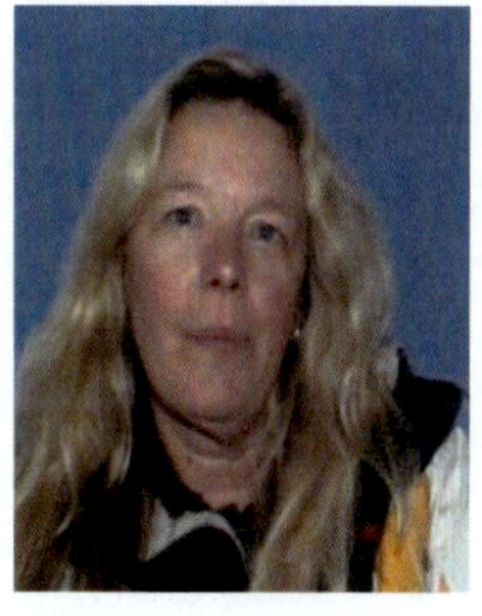

Doris Gundersen is the Head of Research in Helse Fonna, which is a region on the west coast of Norway consisting of four hospitals. She completed her PhD in 1991 at Weill Cornell Medical College in New York City in the field of epithelial polarity. She then moved to Switzerland and was employed as a researcher in the laboratory of the CPO (Centre Plurudisciplinaire D'Oncologie) at ISREC. Her research was focused on the interaction between T-lymphocytes and tenascin-C. She published several papers in this area. Currently, she is engaged in developing clinical research in Helse-Fonna. In the last few years she has also been involved in research projects dealing with a biological approach to irritable bowel syndrome, and has several publications in this field.

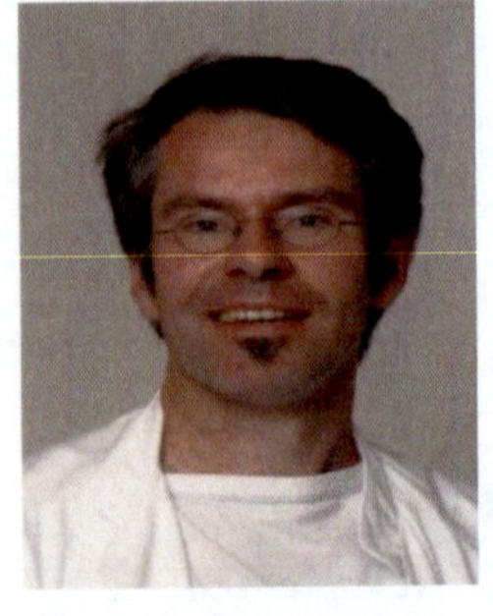

Jan Gunnar Hatlebakk is consultant in gastroenterology at Haukeland University Hospital, and professor of gastroenterology, hepatology and clinical nutrition at University of Bergen Medical School. He was educated at the University of Bergen, becoming MD in 1984 and PhD in 1997. He completed his clinical training at Haukeland University Hospital under Professor Arnold Berstad and has had postdoctoral research stays at The Graduate Hospital, Philadelphia, and Université de Nantes. His research interests have included functional gastrointestinal disorders as well as gastro-oesophageal reflux and gastrointestinal motility disorders.

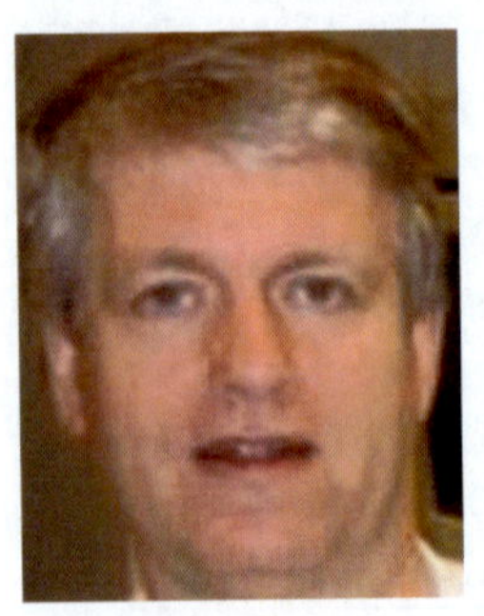

Trygve Hausken is Professor of Gastroenterology and Nutrition, and head of the gastroenterology section, as well as consultant in gastroenterology at Haukeland University Hospital, School of Medicine, University of Bergen, Norway. He completed his PhD (Medicine) in 1992. He has been a specialist in gastroenterology at Haukeland University Hospital since 1989. He has published 122 papers, 15 invited reviews and 3 book chapters. His research field has been functional gastrointestinal disorders, low-grade inflammation, gastrointestinal motility and gastrointestinal ultrasonography, including nutritional imaging and 3D and 4D ultrasound, from basic science to clinical applications.

Preface

Irritable bowel syndrome (IBS) is a common disorder affecting 5 to 20% of the world's population and is most commonly diagnosed in patients younger than 50 years of age, i.e., in the most productive phase of their lives. Irritable bowel syndrome considerably reduces a patient's quality of life and may lead to social isolation, quitting work and broken relationships. Irritable bowel syndrome patients consume a huge amount of health-care resources and are an economic burden to society by being unproductive and consuming welfare resources. Yet IBS patients are dissatisfied with the healthcare providers and welfare officials. They feel that they are misunderstood and regarded as hypochondriacs or mentally ill. Why are these patients met in the healthcare system with a different attitude than other categories of gastrointestinal patients? Is it because IBS is not known to be associated with the development of serious disease or with excess mortality? Is it because we do not understand the pathogenesis? Is it because we lack an effective treatment? Or is it due to the deeply rooted doctrine that we, the physician, have been taught during our education and clinical training, that there is nothing physically wrong with IBS patients and that they occupy our time and use healthcare resources without any improvement?

During the last decade, rapid progress has been made in our understanding of IBS and evidence of a biological cause of IBS has been accumulated. Research to establish treatment for IBS has been intensified and attitudes toward IBS patients are slowly changing. The present book is an attempt to account for this progress and to accelerate the change in attitude of healthcare providers and welfare officials toward IBS patients.

Chapter I

The Maestro, The Artist, The Administrator and The Student

Abstract

The maestro, the artist, the administrator and the student are patients with irritable bowel syndrome (IBS). Their histories, which are based on their medical records and reviews with the patients, illustrate several aspects of IBS. These patients are younger than 50 years of age, in the productive phase of their lives and with families. They feel that they are met with mistrust and neglect by the health-care system. These patients also report that stress aggravates pre-existing symptoms, but does not cause the onset of symptoms. They also show that some IBS patients are subjected to repeated, extensive investigations whereas others are never referred to a gastroenterologist and that whilst some are given an incorrect somatic diagnosis, some are given a psychiatric diagnosis, whereas others undergo unnecessary surgical operations. When irritable bowel syndrome occurs in youths it can prevent their development and integration into society and cause them to become uneducated, inactive and beaten individuals.

The following is a description of four patients with IBS based on their medical records and an interview of about 30 minutes each.

1.1. The Maestro

The maestro is a 40-year-old man, married with four children. He is a well-known music conductor and composer. He is a non-smoker and is not on any medication. He has not been subjected to sexual or physical abuse. Over the years he has suffered from abdominal pain, distension and periods of diarrhoea. He has not sought medical care in all these years. During the last 2 years, in association with an increase in his workload, his abdominal pain and diarrhoea accentuated. He consulted his GP, who referred him to the hospital. At the hospital he underwent an appendectomy under the belief that he was suffering from appendicitis. The excised appendix was completely normal. He continued to suffer from recurrent severe abdominal pain and diarrhoea.

1.2. The Artist

The artist is a 44-year-old woman, married and has three children. She is a well-known painter with an international reputation. She is a non-smoker and is not on any medication. She has not been subjected to sexual or physical abuse. Throughout her whole life she has suffered from periods of abdominal pain, distension and alternating diarrhoea and constipation. At the age of 35, she had abdominal pain almost every day. She consulted her GP, who dismissed her and asked her to come back when she was in pain. She felt that her complaints had not been treated seriously and did not contact another health-care provider until 9 years later. In connection with an assignment as a leader for a gallery, with all the stress it brought, she became much worse and sought health-care. She has undergone extensive neurological and psychological investigations and received a diagnosis of neurasthenia and depression. She continued to suffer from her abdominal symptoms to such a degree that she had to resign from her job at the gallery.

1.3. The Administrator

The administrator is a 40-year-old government employee in a key position. He is married and has two children. He is a smoker and had an allergy diagnosed at the age of 9 years. He uses allergy medication on demand. He has not been subjected to sexual or physical abuse. He has suffered from abdominal pain, distension and alternating diarrhoea and constipation for as long as he can remember. At the age of 24, he had a severe abdominal pain that resulted in hospital admission. Colonoscopy showed a few macroscopic mucosal colonic erythemata. Histopathological examination of biopsies from these areas revealed "non-specific" inflammation. The endoscopic finding of regional mucosal erythemata and the histopathological observation of "non-specific" inflammation, as well unexplained severe abdominal pain, were considered to be enough grounds for a diagnosis of Crohn's disease. He has been treated with high dose steroids without any effect. He experienced severe side effects during this treatment. He continued to have recurrent abdominal pain despite several trials with steroids and 5-ASA. Trials with infliximab infusion and adalimumab injections resulted in anaphylactic shock. During this period, the patient was referred to a university hospital clinic several times. He has undergone several gastroscopies and colonoscopies, four CT and three MR-scans, a capsule endoscopy and a double-balloon enteroscopy. These examinations showed no small bowel stenosis or any sign of present or previous inflammation. Gastroenterologists at the university hospital clinic expressed their doubts about the diagnosis of Crohn's disease, but did not discard it or offer an alternative diagnosis. On one occasion when the patient was in severe pain he was offered an explorative surgery, but he declined. He continued to have recurrent abdominal pain, distension and alternating diarrhoea and constipation. The patient describes the 16 years after being diagnosed with Crohn's disease as living hell. He felt helpless and uncertain, with long periods spent in and out of hospital. He has not been able to have long-term plans for his life and his family. During his periods of hospitalization his wife, who works fulltime, had to take care of their children alone and suffered depression in the belief that her husband was going to die. He lived in fear of being unable to work and the plans for his family were based on the notion that they should be able to manage with his wife's income alone. He looked upon health-care with mistrust and disappointment. Despite all these setbacks, he managed to stay on the top of his profession and advanced in his career.

1.4. The Student

The student is a 22-year-old woman. She is single and a smoker. She has not been subjected to physical or sexual abuse. As far as she can remember she has suffered from attacks of abdominal pain, diarrhoea and urgency, as well as abdominal distension and flatulence. She has seen several GPs, which she changed often because she felt that she was not understood or met with sympathy. She has been treated with an antispasmodic drug without any effect. She used loperamide to control the diarrhoea with considerable success. She reported feeling dirty and smelling bad. She could not socialize with others because she would often have to run to the toilet because of flatulence and diarrhoea. She had a few boyfriends but she could not establish a permanent relationship. She had no friends her own age because she could not share their activities and they got tired of hearing about her health problems. She did well throughout secondary school and moved to the capital to study at a law school. Despite her social isolation and suffering from deep depression, for which she was treated with a tricyclic antidepressant, she did very well in the first year at school and achieved high grades. She was referred to a specialist, who performed gastroscopy and colonoscopy, as well as an abdominal ultrasound examination. He concluded that there was no somatic cause for her symptoms and that she had a functional disorder, which would be better taken care of in primary health-care. During the second year of her studies she could not attend lectures or exams as she had to keep rushing to the toilet because of diarrhoea or flatulence. Loperamide did not help anymore; she could not adjust the dosage. When she took small dose she suffered from diarrhoea and when she took a larger dose she had constipation with increased abdominal pain and flatulence. She had to quit her studies and return home. She tried several jobs, but could not perform well because of the same reasons that caused her to quit her studies. She become more and more socially isolated and seldom left her apartment. She has no income and lives on welfare support.

1.5. Comments

These four patients illustrate several aspects of the whole IBS patient population. They are younger than 50 years of age, in the productive phase of their lives and with families [1-13]. These patients also show that stress aggravates pre-existing symptoms, but does not cause the onset of symptoms. Some IBS patients are subjected to repeated extensive investigations, whilst others are never referred to a gastroenterologist; some receive incorrect somatic diagnoses, some receive a psychiatric diagnosis, whilst others are subjected to unnecessary surgeries. Moreover, it is not unusual for IBS patients to feel that their complaints are not being taken seriously by the health-care provider [14].

The maestro underwent an unnecessary appendectomy. Compared to ulcerative colitis patients, the appendectomy rate in IBS patients is more than four times greater [15]. This high rate of negative appendectomy has been attributed to the atypical presentation of symptoms and the low rate of CT scan usage by physicians [16]. In general, IBS patients have three-fold higher rates of cholecystectomy, two-fold higher rates of appendectomy and hysterectomy, and higher rates of back surgery than examinees without IBS [17-19].

It is not unusual for IBS patients to be given psychiatric diagnoses, even though psychological features correlate poorly with actual symptoms [20]. The artist has been diagnosed with depression and neurasthenia, and she has certainly fulfilled the criteria for both diagnoses. Considering the circumstances described above, it is no wonder that she suffered from reactive depression. With regards to neurasthenia, one should consider this a little further. The term neurasthenia was coined by the psychiatrist George Beard in 1879. Neurasthenia, according to him, is caused by the feverish lifestyle of the New World (America), with an excess of daily activity and energy, and is thus in contrast with the spleen and melancholia of idlers. The syndrome is chronic with both somatic and mental symptoms such as fatigue, back pain, dyspepsia, flatulence, constipation, dysuria, insomnia, sadness, lack of interest and the impoverishment of sexual activity [21-23]. It turned out that neurasthenia was not just a New World syndrome but also an Old World one. Freud used this term with a rather restricted definition, where he retained the somatic symptoms and impoverishment of sexual activity [24]. Freud considered neurasthenia as a defence neurosis with a symptomatology that is not a symbolic and overdetermined expression and for which the aetiology must not be sought in childhood conflicts but in a present frustration [24]. Considering Freud's definition of neurasthenia, this diagnosis would fit almost all IBS patients seeking health-care.

It is not unusual for a bowel preparation with a colonic cleansing agent for colonoscopy to induce macroscopic mucosal colonic erythema. Biopsies from these areas show non-specific inflammation. Furthermore, oral sodium phosphate is being increasingly used as a colonic agent for colonoscopy. In Norway, sodium phosphate is widely used because it is effective and well tolerated. Unfortunately, sodium phosphate induces non-specific aphthoid-like mucosal lesions in the rectum, colon and terminal ileum (Figure 1) [25-27]. Biopsies from these lesions show non-specific inflammation. Patients who exhibit these endoscopic lesions do not develop any clinical signs of Crohn's disease (unpublished data). Although these lesions resemble those seen in Crohn's disease, they are smaller and more superficial. A combination of low-volume polyethylene glycol [PEG) with bisacodyl is now commonly used for colon cleansing [28, 29]. However, we found that this combination induces colonic mucosal lesions in some patients [Figure 2). Biopsies from these lesions revealed non-specific inflammation (unpublished data). Polyethylene glycol has not been shown to alter the histological features of the colonic mucosa [29]. When taken in conjunction with bisacodyl, however, PEG has been associated with colonic ischaemia [30]. Irritable bowel syndrome patients with recurrent severe abdominal pain and diarrhoea, such as the administrator, and with colonic lesions induced by cleansing agents are at risk of being diagnosed with Crohn's disease.

Irritable bowel syndrome affecting individuals of a young age, who comprise a considerable proportion of the IBS population, can lead to impairments in personal development and social isolation, preventing them from receiving an education and gaining work. Thus, IBS in adolescence can transform a young, promising individual with a potentially reproductive life, such as in the case of the student, into an inactive and beaten person who is a burden to society.

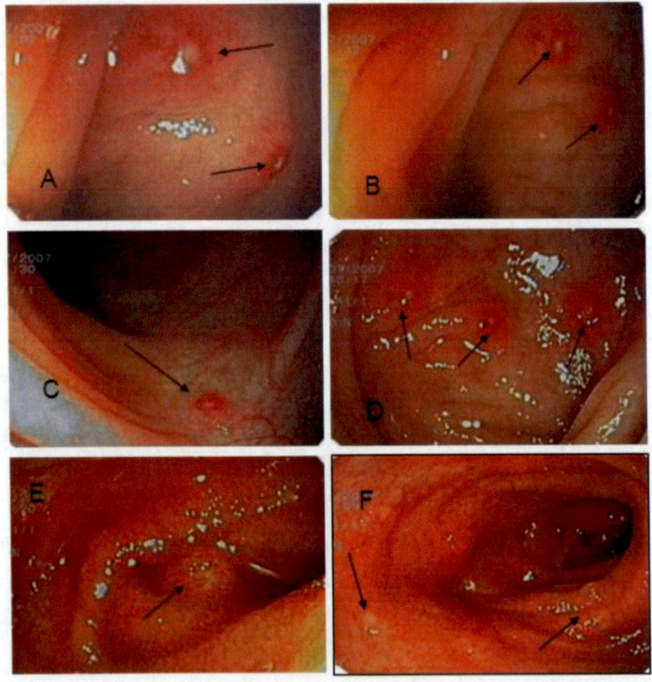

Figure 1. Colon cleansing agent sodium phosphate-induced non-specific aphthoid-like mucosal lesions in the rectum (A and B), colon (C and D) and terminal ileum (E and F).

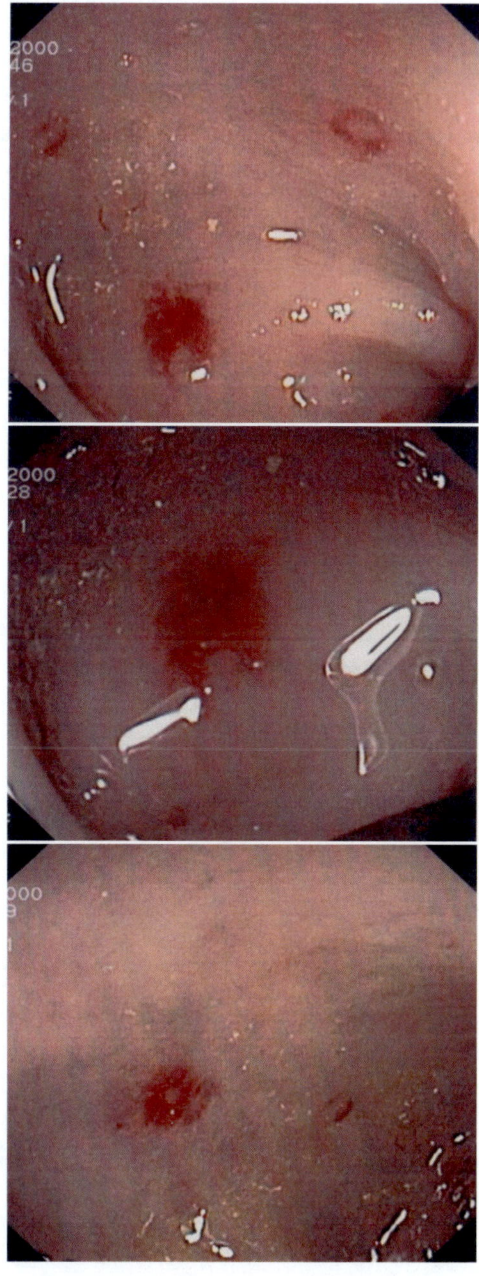

Figure 2. Colonic mucosal lesions induced by the combination of low volume polyethylene glycol (PEG) with bisacodyl used for colon cleansing.

References

[1]   Agreus L, Svarsudd K, Nygren O, Tibblin G. Irritable bowel syndrome and dyspepsia in general population: overlap and lack of stability over time. *Gastroenterology* 1995; 109: 671-680.

[2]   Thompson WG, Haeton KW. Functional bowel disorders in apparently healthy people. *Gastorenterology* 1980; 79: 283-288.

[3]   Kennedy TM, Jones RH, Hungin AP, O'Flanagan H, Kelly P. Irritable bowel syndrome, gastro-oesophageal reflux, and bronchial hyper-responsiveness in the general population. *Gut* 1998; 43: 770-774.

[4]   Drossman DA, Li Z, Andruzzi E, Temple RD, Talley NJ, Thompson WG, Whitehead WE, Janssens J, P Funch-Jensen , E Corazziari . U.S. householder survey of functional gastrointestinal disorders. Prevalence, sociodemography, and health impact. *Dig Dis Sci* 1993; 38: 1569-1580.

[5]   Talley NJ, Gabriel SE, Harmsen WS, Zinsmeister AR, Evans RW. Medical costs in community subjects with irritable bowel syndrome. *Gastroenterology* 1995; 109: 1736-1741.

[6]   Hugin AP, Whonwell PJ, Tack J, Mearin F. The prevalence, patterns and impact of irritable bowel syndrome: an international survey of 40,000 subjects. *Alment Pharmacol Ther* 2003; 17: 643-650.

[7]   Jones R, Lydeard S. Irritable bowel syndrome in the general population. *BMJ* 1992; 304: 87-90.

[8]   Bordie AK. Functional disorders of the colon. *J Indian Med Assoc* 1972; 58: 451-456.

[9]   O`Keefe EA, Talley NJ, Zinsmeister AR, Jacobsen SJ. Bowel disorders impair functional status and quality of life in the elderly: a population-based study. *J Biol Sci Med Sci* 1995; 50: M184-M189.

[10]   Everhart JE, Renault PF. Irritable bowel syndrome in office-based practice in the United States. Gastroenterology 1991; 100: 998-1005.

[11]   Wilson S, Roberts L, Roalfe A, Bridge P, Sukhdev S. Prevalence of irritable bowel syndrome: a community survey. *Br J Gen Pract* 2004; 54: 495-502.

[12]   Harvey RF, Salih SY, Read AE. Organic and functional disorders in 2000 gastroenterology outpatients. *Lancet* 1983; 1: 632-634.

[13]   Spiegel BM. The burden of IBS: looking at metrics. *Curr Gastroenterol Rep* 2009; 11: 265-269.

[14]   Dancy CP, Backhouse S. Towards a better understanding of patients with irritable bowel syndrome. *J Adv Nurs* 1993; 18: 1443-1450.

[15] Burns DG. The risk of abdominal surgery in irritable bowel syndrome. *S Afr Med J* 1986; 70: 91.

[16] Lu CL, Liu CC, Fuh JL, Liu PY, Wu CW, Chang FY, Lee SD. Irritable bowel syndrome and negative appendectomy: a prospective multivariable investigation. *Gut* 2007; 56: 655-660.

[17] Longstreth GF, Yao JE. Irritable bowel syndrome and surgery: a multivariable analysis. *Gastroenterology* 2004; 126: 1665-1673.

[18] Cole JA, Yeaw JM, Cutone JA, Kuo B, Huang Z, Earnest DL, Walker AM. The incidence of abdominal and pelvic surgery among patients with irritable bowel syndrome. *Dig Dis Sci* 2005; 50: 2268-2275.

[19] Corazziari E, Attili AF, Angeletti C, De Santis A. Gallstones, cholecystectomy and irritable bowel syndrome [IBS] MICOL population-based study. Dig Liver Dis 2008; 40: 944-950.

[20] Spiller RC. Treatment of irritable bowel syndrome. *Current Treatment Options in Gastroenterology*, 2003; 6: 329-337.

[21] Beard G. Neurasthenia as a cause of inebriety. New York: E. B. Treat 1879.

[22] Beard G. American nervousness: Its causes and consequences. New York: E. B. Treat 1881.

[23] Beard G. Sexual neurasthenia [nervous exhaustion), its hygiene, causes, symptoms and treatment. New York: E. B. Treat 1884.

[24] Freud S. On the grounds for detaching a particular syndrome from neurasthenia under the description "anxiety neurosis." SE 1894; 3: 85-115.

[25] Zwas FR, Cirillo NW, el-Serag HB, Eisen RN. Colonic mucosal abnormalities associated with oral sodium phosphate solution. *Gastrointest Endosc* 1996; 43: 463-466.

[26] Chiumska A, Bebes Z, Mukensnabl P, Zamecnik M. Histologic findings after sodium phosphate bowel preparation for colonoscopy. *Cesk Patol* 2010; 46: 37-41.

[27] Adamcewicz M, Bearelly D, Porat G, Friedenberg FK. Mechanism of action and toxicities of purgatives used for colonoscopy preparation. *Expert Opin Drug Met Toxiol* 2011; 7: 89-101.

[28] Adams WJ, Meagher AP, Lubowski DZ, King DW. Bisacodyl reduces the volume of polyethylene glycol solution required for bowel preparation. *Dis Colon Rectum* 1994; 37: 229-233.

[29] DiPalma JA, Wolff BG, Meagher A, Cleveland M. Comparison of reduced volume versus four liters sulfate-free electrolyte lavage

solutions for colonoscopy colon cleansing. *Am J Gastroenterol* 2003; 98: 2187-2191.

[30] Baudet JS, Castro V, Redondo I. Recurrent ischemic colitis induced by colonoscopy bowel lavage. *Am J Gastroenterol* 2010; 105: 700–701.

Chapter II

Symptoms, Incidence and Prevalence

Abstract

Irritable bowel syndrome (IBS) is a common chronic disorder with a prevalence ranging from 5 to 20% of the world's population. The annual incidence of IBS is between 196 and 260 per 100,000. Irritable bowel syndrome is more common in women than in men, and is more commonly diagnosed in patients younger than 50 years of age. This condition is characterised by abdominal discomfort or pain, altered bowel habits, and often bloating and abdominal distension. The degree of symptoms varies in different patients from tolerable to severe. Also, the time pattern and discomfort varies immensely from patient to patient. Some complain of daily symptoms, while others report intermittent symptoms at intervals of weeks/months. Irritable bowel syndrome reduces quality of life with the same degree of impairment as major chronic diseases such as diabetes, congestive heart failure, renal insufficiency, hepatic cirrhosis and inflammatory bowel diseases and the economic burden on the health care system and society is high. However, IBS is not known to be associated with the development of serious disease or with excess mortality. Conventional therapy for IBS has focused on the systematic relief of symptoms such as pain, diarrhoea or constipation.

Irritable bowel syndrome (IBS) affects as many as 12-46% of the adult population and this large variation can be explained by the use of different delimitations in different studies [1, 2]. However, recent diagnostic criteria, such as Rome criteria I, II or III, suggest that the IBS affects 5 to 20% of individuals worldwide (Figure 3) [3-32]. The annual incidence of IBS in USA is 196 and in UK 260 per 100 000 [33, 34]. This can be compared with the annual incidence of colon cancer (50 per 100 000) and IBD (10 per 10000) [35, 36]. It is worth noting, however, that this incidence of IBS is based on people who sought medical care and it is well known that people may have IBS symptom and are not seeking care [37]. IBS is more common in women than in men, with as many as twice the number of females as males affected and more commonly diagnosed in patients younger than 50 years of age [5,15,38-48]. It has been claimed that men with IBS exhibit less male characteristics, but there is not, however, any difference in the prevalence of homosexuality between patients and controls [49].

IBS symptoms range from diarrhoea to constipation or a combination of the two, coupled with severe abdominal pain or discomfort as well as abdominal distension (Figure 4) [1]. The degree of symptoms varies in different patients from tolerable to severe, where the experience of pain may be experienced as a nagging, colicky, sharp or dull feeling of pain. Also, the time pattern and discomfort varies immensely from patient to patient [5,15, 38-48]. Some complain of daily symptoms, while others report intermittent symptoms at intervals of weeks/months.

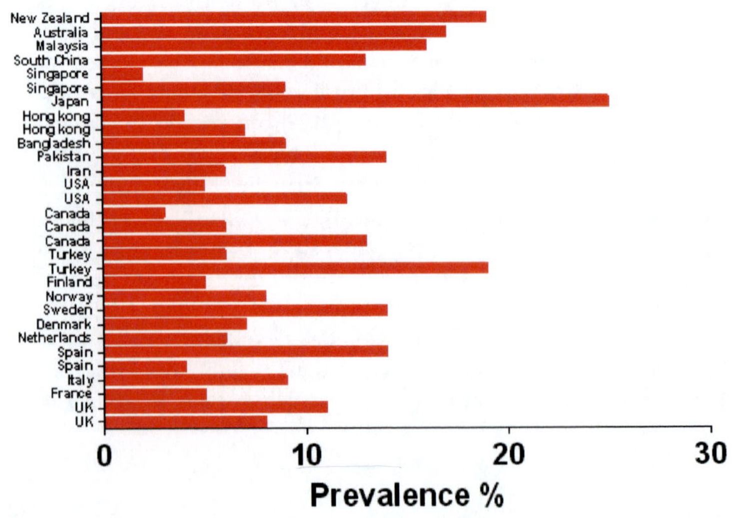

Figure 3. The prevalence of IBS according to Rome criteria in different countries.

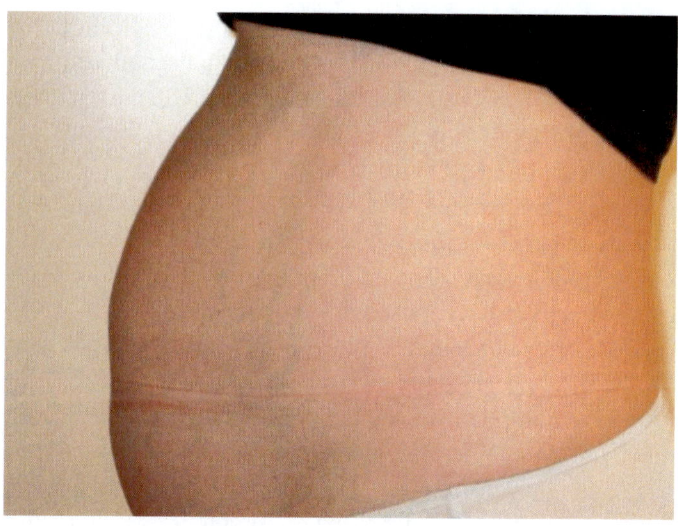

Figure 4. Abdominal distension in a female patient with IBS.

IBS causes reduced quality of life to the same degree of impairment as major chronic diseases such as diabetes, congestive heart failure, renal insufficiency and hepatic cirrhosis [50-54]. In an international survey of patients with IBS [55], patients with IBS reported impaired health status (restricting on average 73 days of activity in a year), poor health-related quality of life (particularly with dietary restrictions), mood disturbance, and interference with daily activity. Astonishingly, and illustrating the psychological toll of the condition, this survey showed that IBS patients would give up 25% of their remaining life (average 15 years) and 14% would risk a 1/1000 chance of death to receive a treatment that would make them symptom-free. IBS is not known, however, to be associated with development of serious disease or with excess mortality [56, 57].

Although a minority (10-50%) of IBS patients seeks healthcare, they generate a substantial workload in both primary and secondary care [58-60]. It seems that there is a racial and cultural difference in healthcare-seeking behaviour. Thus, Hispanics are less likely than non-Hispanic whites to seek health-care for bowel complaints and Hispanics are also more likely to self-medicate with folk remedies to maintain good bowel function [61]. It is estimated that 12-14% of primary care patient visits and 28% of referrals to gastroenterologists are IBS patients, making this a more common reason for a visit to a physician than diabetes, hypertension or asthma [40, 47, 62-63]. Not only do IBS patients visit their doctors more frequently, but more diagnostic tests are also performed, and they consume more medications, miss more workdays, have lower work productivity, are hospitalised more frequently, and incur more overall direct costs than those without IBS [40, 47, 62-63]. The annual costs in USA (both direct and indirect) to manage patients with IBS are estimated at 15-30 billion USD [40, 47, 62-63].

Conventional therapy for IBS has focused on systematic relief of symptoms such as pain, diarrhoea or constipation. Evidence of the long-term benefit of pharmacological agents has been sparse and new agents, which proved to be effective, have raised issues concerning safety [64, 65]. Not surprisingly, alternative therapies have been considered. Thus, cognitive behavioural therapy and gut-directed hypnotherapy have been used with good results [66]. Other non-pharmacological approaches have been also tried with proven effect on symptoms and quality of life in patients with IBS [67]. Reassurance and information to patients with IBS [67,68,70], dietary management [69,70], the administration of probiotics, and regular exercise have all been found to reduce symptoms and improve quality of life of IBS patients [71-73].

References

[1]   Systematic review on the management of irritable bowel syndrome in the European Union. *Eur J Gastroenterol Hepatol* 2007; 19 (Supp 1): 11-37.

[2]   Thompson WG. A world view of IBS. In Camilleri M, Spiller R Eds., Irritable bowel syndrome: Diagnosis and treatment. Saunders, Philadelphia and London, 2002; pp. 17-26.

[3]   Quigley EM, Locke GR, Mueller-Lissner S, Paulo LG, Tytgat GN, Helfrich I, Schaefer E. Prevalence and management of abdominal cramping and pain: a multinational survey. *Aliment Pharmacol Ther* 2006; 24: 411-419.

[4]   Vandvik PO, Lydersen S, Farup PG. Prevalence, comorbidity and impact of irritable bowel syndrome in Norway. *Scand J Gastroenterol* 2006; 41: 650-656.

[5]   Drossman DA, Li Z, Andruzzi E, Temple RD, Talley NJ, Thompson WG, Whitehead WE, Janssens J, Funch-Jensen P, Corazziari E, et al. US householder survey of functional gastrointestinal disorders. Prevalence, sociodemography, and health impact. *Dig Dis Sci* 1993; 38: 1569-1580.

[6] Saito YA, Talley NJ, Melton J, Fett S, Zinsmeister AR, Locke GR. The effect of new diagnostic criteria for irritable bowel syndrome on community prevalence estimates. *Neurogastroenterol Motil* 2003; 15: 687-694.

[7] Thompson WG, Irvine EJ, Pare P, Ferrazzi S, Rance L. Functional gastrointestinal disorders in Canada: first population-based survey using Rome II criteria with suggestions for improving the questionnaire. *Dig Dis Sci* 2002; 47: 225-235.

[8] Li FX, Patten SB, Hilsden RJ, Sutherland LR. Irritable bowel syndrome and health-related quality of life: a population-based study in Calgary, Alberta. *Can J Gastroenterol* 2003; 17: 259-263.

[9] Boyce PM, Koloski NA, Talley NJ. Irritable bowel syndrome according to varying diagnostic criteria: are the new Rome II criteria unnecessarily restrictive for research and practice? *Am J Gastroenterol* 2000; 95: 3176-383.

[10] Barbezat G, Poulton R, Milne B, Howell S, Fawcett JP, Talley N. Prevalence and correlates of irritable bowel symptoms in a New Zealand birth cohort. *NZ Med J* 2002; 115: U220.

[11] Boekema PJ, van Dam van Isselt EF, Bots ML, Smout AJ. Functional bowel symptoms in a general Dutch population and associations with common stimulants. *Neth J Med* 2001; 59: 23-30.

[12] Mearin F, Badia X, Balboa A, Baró E, Caldwell E, Cucala M, Díaz-Rubio M, Fueyo A, Ponce J, Roset M, Talley NJ. Irritable bowel syndrome prevalence varies enormously depending on the employed diagnostic criteria: comparison of Rome II versus previous criteria in a general population. *Scand J Gastroenterol* 2001; 36: 1155-1161.

[13] Gaburri M, Bassotti G, Bacci G, Cinti A, Bosso R, Ceccarelli P, Paolocci N, Pelli MA, Morelli A. Functional gut disorders and health care seeking behavior in an Italian non-patient population. *Recenti Prog Med* 1989; 80: 241–244.

[14] Coffin B, Dapoigny M, Cloarec D, Comet D, Dyard F. Relationship between severity of symptoms and quality of life in 858 patients with irritable bowel syndrome. *Gastroenterol Clin Biol* 2004; 28: 11–15.

[15] Agreus L, Svarsudd K, Nygren O, Tibblin G. Irritable bowel syndrome and dyspepsia in general population: overlap and lack of stability over time. *Gastroenterology* 1995; 109: 671-680.

[16] Hillila MT, Farkkila MA. Prevalence of irritable bowel syndrome according to different diagnostic criteria in a non-selected adult population. *Aliment Pharmacol Ther* 2004; 20: 339–345.

[17] Kay L, Jorgensen T, Jensen KH. The epidemiology of irritable bowel syndrome in a random population: prevalence, incidence, natural history and risk factors. *J Intern Med* 1994; 236: 23–30.

[18] Hoseini-Asl MK, Amra B. Prevalence of irritable bowel syndrome in Shahrekord, Iran. *Indian J Gastroenterol* 2003; 22: 215–216.

[19] Karaman N, Turkay C, Yonem O. Irritable bowel syndrome prevalence in city center of Sivas. *Turk J Gastroenterol* 2003; 14: 128–131.

[20] Celebi S, Acik Y, Deveci SE, et al. Epidemiological features of irritable bowel syndrome in a Turkish urban society. *J Gastroenterol Hepatol* 2004; 19: 738–743.

[21] Masud MA, Hasan M, Khan AK. Irritable bowel syndrome in a rural community in Bangladesh: prevalence, symptoms pattern, and health care seeking behavior. *Am J Gastroenterol* 2001; 96: 1547–5152.

[22] Huerta I, Valdovinos MA, Schmulson M. Irritable bowel syndrome in Mexico. *Dig Dis* 2001; 19: 251–257.

[23] Kwan AC, Hu WH, Chan YK, et al. Prevalence of irritable bowel syndrome in Hong Kong. *J Gastroenterol Hepatol* 2002; 17: 1180–1186.

[24] Lau EM, Chan FK, Ziea ET, et al. Epidemiology of irritable bowel syndrome in Chinese. *Dig Dis Sci* 2002; 47: 2621–2624.

[25] Schlemper R, Van der Werf SJ, Vandenbroucke JP, et al. Peptic ulcer, non-ulcer dyspepsia and irritable bowel syndrome in The Netherlands and Japan. *Scand J Gastroenterol Suppl* 1993; 28: 33–41.

[26] Ho KY, Kang JY, Seow A. Prevalence of gastrointestinal symptoms in a multiracial Asian population, with particular reference to reflux-type symptoms. *Am J Gastroenterol* 1998; 93: 1816–1822.

[27] Xiong LS, Chen MH, Chen HX, et al. A population-based epidemiologic study of irritable bowel syndrome in South China: stratified randomized study by cluster's sampling. *Aliment Pharmacol Ther* 2004; 19: 1217–1224.

[28] Gwee KA, Wee S, Wong ML, et al. The prevalence, symptom characteristics, and impact of irritable bowel syndrome in an Asian urban community. *Am J Gastroenterol* 2004; 99:924–31.

[29] Rajendra S, Alahuddin S. Prevalence of irritable bowel syndrome in a multiethnic Asian population. *Aliment Pharmacol Ther* 2004; 19: 704–706.

[30] Jafri W, Yakoob J, Jafri N Islam M, Ali QM. "Irritable bowel syndrome and health seeking behaviour in different communities of Pakistan". *J Pak Med Assoc* 2007; 57: 285–287.

[31] Jafri W, Yakoob J, Jafri N, Islam M, Ali QM. Frequency of irritable bowel syndrome in college students. *J Ayub Med Coll Abbottabad* 2005; 4: 9–11.

[32] Boivin M. Socioeconomic impact of irritable bowel syndrome in Canada. *Can. J. Gastroenterol* 2001; 15 (Suppl B): 8B–11B.

[33] Locke III GR, Yawn B, Wollan PC, Melton III LJ, Lydick E, Talley NJ. Incidence of clinical diagnosis of irritable bowel syndrome in a united states population. *Aliment Pharmacol Ther* 2004; 19: 1025-1031.

[34] Rodriguez G, Ruigomez LA, Wallander MA, Johansson S, Olbe L. Detection of colorectal tumor and infalammatory bowel disease during follow-up of patients with intial dignosis of irritable bowel syndrome. *Scand J Gastroenterol* 2000; 35: 306-311.

[35] Rex DK. Rational for colonoscopy screening and estimated effectiveness in clinical practice. *Gastrointest Endosc Clin N Am* 2002; 12: 65-75.

[36] Loftus EV JR, Schoenfeld P, Sandborn WJ. The epidemiology and natural history of Cohn's disease in population-based patient cohorts from North America: a systematic review. *Aliment Pharmacol Ther* 2002; 16: 51-60.

[37] Koloski NA, Talley NJ, Boyce PM. Predictors of health care seeking for irritable bowel syndrome and nonulcer dyspepsia: a critical review of the literature on symptom and psychosocial factors. *Am J Gastroenterol* 2001: 96: 1340-1349.

[38] Thompson WG, Haeton KW. Functional bowel disorders in apparently healthy people. *Gastorenterology* 1980; 79: 283-288.

[39] Kennedy TM, Jones RH, Hungin AP, O'Flanagan H, Kelly P. Irritable bowel syndrome, gastro-oesophageal reflux, and bronchial hyper-responsiveness in the general population. *Gut* 1998; 43: 770-774.

[40] Talley NJ, Gabriel SE, Harmsen WS, Zinsmeister AR, Evans RW. Medical costs in community subjects with irritable bowel syndrome. *Gastroenterology* 1995; 109: 1736-1741.

[41] Hugin AP, Whonwell PJ, Tack J, Mearin F. The prevalence, patterns and impact of irritable bowel syndrome: an international survey of 40,000 subjects. *Alment Pharmacol Ther* 2003; 17: 643-650.

[42] Jones R, Lydeard S. Irritable bowel syndrome in the general population. *BMJ* 1992; 304: 87-90.

[43] Bordie AK. Functional disorders of the colon. *J Indian Med Assoc* 1972; 58: 451-456.

[44] O`Keefe EA, Talley NJ, Zinsmeister AR, Jacobsen SJ. Bowel disorders impair functional status and quality of life in the elderly: a population-based study. *J Biol Sci Med Sci* 1995; 50: M184-M189.

[45] Everhart JE, Renault PF Irritable bowel syndrome in office-based practice in the United States. *Gastroenterology* 1991; 100: 998-1005.

[46] Wilson S, Roberts L, Roalfe A, Bridge P, Sukhdev S. Prevalence of irritable bowel syndrome: a community survey. *Br J Gen Pract* 2004; 54: 495-502.

[47] Harvey RF, Salih SY, Read AE. Organic and functional disorders in 2000 gastroenterology outpatients. *Lancet* 1983; 1: 632-634.

[48] Spiegel BM. The burden of IBS: looking at metrics. *Curr Gastroenterol Rep* 2009; 11: 265-269.

[49] Miller V, Whitaker K, Morris JA, Whorwell PJ. Gender and irritable bowel syndrome.: in male connection. *J Clin Gastroenterol* 2004; 38: 558-580.

[50] Whitehead WE, Burnett CK, Cook EW,III, Taub E. Impact of irritable bowel syndrome on quality of life. *Dig Dig Sci* 1996; 41: 2248-2253.

[51] Gralnek IM, Hays RD, Kilbourne A, Naliboff B, Mayer EA. The impact of irritable bowel syndrome on health related quality of life. *Gastroenterology* 2000; 11: 654-660.

[52] Huerta-Icelo I, Hinojosa C, Santa Maria A, Schmulson M. Diferencias en la calidad de vida (CV) entre pacientes con sindrome de Intestino irritable (SII) y la poblacon mexicana evaluadas mediante el SF-36. *Rev Mex Gastroenterol* 2001; 66 (Suppl 2): 145-146.

[53] Schmulson M, Robles G, Kershenobich, Lopez-Ridaura R, Hinojosa C, Durate A. Los pacientes con trastornos funcionales digestivos (TFD) tienen major compromiso de la calidad de vida (CV) evaluadas por el SF-36 comparados con pacientes con hepatitis C y pancreatitis cronica. *Rev Mex Gastroenterol* 2000; 65 (Suppl-Resumenes): 50-51.

[54] Pace F, Molteni P, Bollani S, Sarzi-Puttini P, Stockbrügger R, Biani Porro G, Drossman DA. Inflammatory bowel diseases versus irritable bowel syndrome: a hospital-based control study of disease impact on quality of life. *Scand J Gastroenterol* 2003; 38: 1031-1038.

[55] Drossman DA, Morris CB, Schneck S, Hu YJ, Norton NJ, Norton WF, Weinland SR, Dalton C, Leserman J, Bangdiwala SI. International survey of patients with IBS: symptom features and their severity, health status, treatments, and risk taking to achieve clinical benefit. *J Clin Gastroenterol* 2009; 43: 541-550.

[56] Sloth H, Jorgensen LS. Chronic non-organic upper abdominal pain: diagnostic safety and prognosis of gastrointestinal and non-intestinal symptoms. A 5-to 7-year follow-up study. *Scand J Gastroenterol* 1988; 23: 1275-1280.

[57] Harvey RF, Mauad EC, Brown MA. Prognosis in irritable bowel syndrome: a 5-year prospective study. *Lancet* 1987; i: 963-965.

[58] Schuster MM. Defining and diagnosing irritable bowel syndrome. *Am J Manag Care* 2001; 7: S246-251.

[59] National ambulatory Medical Care Survey. National Center for Health Statistics: NAMCS Description. Available at: http://www.cdc.gov/nchs/about/major/ahcd/namcsdes.htm.

[60] Mitchel CM, Drossman DA. Survey of AGA membership relating to patients with functional gastrointestinal disorders. *Gastroenterology* 1987; 92: 1282-1284.

[61] Zuckerman MJ,Guerra LG, Drossman DA, Foland JA, Gregory GG. Health-care-seeking behaviors related to bowel complains. Hispanics versus non-Hispanic whites. *Dig Dis Sci* 1996; 41: 77-82.

[62] American Gastroenterological association. *The Burden of Gastrointestinal Diseases*. 2001.

[63] Sandler RS, Everhart JE, Donowitz M, Adams E, Cronin K, Goodman C, Gemmen E, Shah S, Avdic A, Rubin R. The burden of selected digestive diseases in the United States. *Gastroenterology* 2002; 122: 1500-1511.

[64] Spanier JS, Howden CW, Jones MP. A systematic review of alternative therapies in irritable bowel syndrome. *Arch Intern Med* 2003; 163: 265-274.

[65] Pasricha PJ. Desperately seeking serotonin: a commentary on the withdrawal of tegaserod and the state of functional and motility disorders. *Gastroenterology* 2007; 132: 2287-2290.

[66] Wald A, Rakel D. Behavioural and complementary approaches for the treatment of irritable bowel syndrome. *Nutr Clin Pract* 2008; 23: 284-292.

[67] Schmulson MJ, Ortiz-Garrido OM, Hinojosa C, Arcila D. A single session of reassurance can acutely improve the self-perception of impairment in patients with IBS. *J Psychosom Res* 2006; 6: 461-467.

[68] Clowell LJ, Prather CM, Philips SF, Zinsmeister AR. Effects of an irritable bowel syndrome educational class on health-promoting behaviours and symptoms. *Am J Gastroenterol* 1998; 93: 901-905.

[69] Heizer WD, Southern S, McGovern S. The role of diet in symptoms of irritable bowel syndrome in adults: a narrative review. *J Am Diet Assoc* 2009; 109: 1204-1214.

[70] Singh N, Makharia GK, Joshi YK. Dietary survey and total dietary intake in patients with irritable bowel syndrome attending a tertiary referral hospital. *Indian J Gastroenterol* 2008; 27: 66-70.

[71] Brenner DM, Moeller MJ, Chey WD, Schoenfeld PS. The utility of probiotics in the treatment of irritable bowel syndrome: a systematic review. *Am J Gastroenterol* 2009; 104: 1033-1049.

[72] Spiller R. Review article: probiotics and prebiotics in irritable bowel syndrome. *Alment Pharmacol Ther* 2008; 28: 385-396.

[73] Levy RL, Linde JA, Feld KA, Crowell MD, Jeffery RW. The association of gastrointestinal symptoms with weight diet and exercise in weight-loss program participants. *Clin Gastroenterol Hepatol* 2005; 2: 992-996.

Chapter III

Diagnosis

Abstract

There is no biochemical, histopathological or radiological diagnostic test for IBS. Rather, the diagnosis of IBS is based on symptom assessments such as the Rome III criteria. In addition to these criteria, warning symptoms (red flags) such as age >50 years, a short history of symptoms, nocturnal symptoms, weight loss, rectal bleeding, anaemia and the presence of markers of inflammation or infections should be excluded. Irritable bowel syndrome patients are sub-grouped on the basis of differences in predominant bowel pattern as diarrhoea-predominant (IBS-D), constipation-predominant (IBS-C), or a mixture of both diarrhoea and constipation (IBS-M) and un-subtyped IBS with insufficient abnormality of stool consistency to meet criteria for IBS C, D or M. A wide range of biomarkers for the diagnosis of IBS have been considered, but only gut transit measured by radioisotope markers meets the criteria for reproducibility and availability. However, radioisotope tests are expensive and of limited availability. It has been reported that the density of chromogranin A-containing cells is low in the duodenum and colon of both IBS-constipation and IBS-diarrhoea patients. Duodenal chromogranin A cell density could be used as a histopathological marker for the diagnosis of IBS with 91% sensitivity and 89% specificity. Because of symptom overlap with coeliac disease and inflammatory bowel disease, we suggest that duodenal biopsies or serological tests for coeliac disease and ileo-colonoscopy with biopsies could be used to exclude these diseases.

There is no biochemical, histopathological or radiological diagnostic test for IBS. Rather, the diagnosis of IBS is based on symptom assessment. The first attempt to establish diagnostic criteria for IBS was made by Manning and colleagues, where 109 unselected patients with abdominal pain or change in bowel habit or both were examined (Table 1) [1]. Over the last 15 years, more attention has been paid to IBS, and Rome working parties elaborated detailed, accurate, and clinically useful definitions of the syndrome.

Thus, Rome I criteria [2], II [3] and III [4] have been established (Table 2). In addition to these criteria, warnings symptoms (red flags) such as age >50 years, short history of symptoms, nocturnal symptoms, weight loss, rectal bleeding, anaemia, and the presence of markers for inflammation or infections should be excluded. IBS patients are sub-grouped on the basis of differences in predominant bowel pattern as diarrhoea-predominant (IBS-D), constipation-predominant (IBS-C), or a mixture of both diarrhoea and constipation (IBS-M) and un-subtyped IBS in patients with insufficient abnormality of stool consistency to meet criteria for IBS C, D or M (Table 3). It has been reported that around one third of patients have IBS-D, one third have IBS-C, and the remainder have IBS-M [5-7]. The division of IBS patients into subtypes is useful for clinical practice and symptomatic treatment. In clinical practice, however, it is common that IBS patients switch from one subtype to another over time.

These patients are now called "alternators". More than 75% of IBS patients change to either of the other 2 subtypes at least once over a 1-year period [7].

It has been reported that there are no consistent differences in sensitivity or specificity between Manning, Rome I, and II and that Rome criteria III needs to be tested [8]. In clinical practice, few clinicians in primary- and secondary-care use the Rome criteria systematically, but instead rely more on a holistic approach [9-12].

Table 1. Manning criteria for the diagnosis of Irritable bowel syndrome (IBS)

1. Abdominal pain that is relieved by defecation
2. More frequent and looser stools at onset of pain
4. Visible abdomen distension
5. Passage of mucus per rectum and sense of incomplete evacuation

Table 2. Rome III criteria for the diagnosis of irritable bowel syndrome

Recurrent abdominal pain or discomfort with onset at least 3 months prior to diagnosis, associated with 2 or more of the following, at least 3 days/month in the last 3 months:

1. Improvement with defecation

2. Onset associated with change in frequency of stool

3. Onset associated with change in form (appearance) of stool

Symptoms that cumulatively support the diagnosis are:

* Abnormal stool frequency (greater than 3 bowel movements per day or less than 3 bowels movements per week);

* Abnormal stool form (lump/hard or loose/watery stool);

* Abnormal stool passage (straining, urgency or feeling of incomplete evacuation);

* Passage of mucous;

* Bloating or feeling of abdominal distension

Table 3. Subtyping of Irritable bowel syndrome (IBS)

1) IBS with constipation (IBS-C)-hard or lumpy stools $\geq$25% and loos or watery stools <25% of bowel movements

2) IBS with diarrhea (IBS-D)-loos or watery stools $\geq$25% and hard or lumpy stools <25% of bowel movements

3) Mixed IBS (IBS-M)-loos or watery stools $\geq$25% and hard or lumpy stools $\geq$25% of bowel movements

4) Unsubtyped IBS-insufficient abnormality of stool consistency to meet criteria for IBS-C,D or M

Several gastroenterologists believe that a symptom-based diagnosis, such as that based on the Rome III criteria, without red flags is enough for the diagnosis of IBS and no further investigations are needed. Incorporating red flags to Rome criteria has been found to be highly specific, but not particularly sensitive [13]. The American College of Gastroenterology Task Force does not recommend routine colonic imaging in patients younger than 50 years of age without alarming features and colonoscopic imaging should be reserved for those over the age of 50 years for the purpose of cancer screening [14]. The guidelines of the of The British Society of Gastroenterology go further by recommending an examination of the colon earlier if there is a first degree relative affected by colorectal cancer younger than 45 years, or two first degree relatives [15]. The British Society Of Gastroenterology recommended further more investigation in IBS-D due to the overlap with other diarrhoea diseases such as celiac and inflammatory bowel diseases [15]. These recommendations seem to be suitable for detecting and diagnosing colorectal cancer in this group of patients. In fact, colorectal cancer is the diagnosis that patients fear the most and physicians are most concerned about missing.

It is rather difficult to clinically distinguish IBS from adult-onset celiac disease (CD) [16-22]. In patients with CD presenting in adulthood, minimal or atypical symptoms are often encountered [18, 19, 21]. The breadth of the spectrum of symptoms associated with IBS results in a potential for overlap of IBS and CD symptomatologies. Consequently, individuals with CD presenting with relatively vague abdominal symptoms are at risk of been dismissed as having IBS [23]. The situation is further complicated by the fact that the abdominal symptoms of both IBS and CD patients are triggered by the ingestion of wheat products. In CD patients, this is due to gluten allergy, while in IBS the effect is attributed to the long sugar polymer fructan in the wheat [23]. The prevalence of CD in IBS varies in different studies and varies between 0.04 to 4.7% [21, 22, 24-34]. Regardless of the number of the CD patients among patients diagnosed with IBS, we believe that IBS patients with all subtypes should be routinely screened for CD. This is in line with current opinion in the field [34-37]. Recently, it has been proposed that IBS patients with wheat intolerance and who possess the genotype associated with CD (HLA DQ2 or DR3), but do not have typical serological markers or changes in small intestine histology, exhibit other immunological evidence of gluten reactivity and respond to a gluten-free diet [36,37].

Discriminating inflammatory bowel diseases (IBD) from IBS, especially with mild disease activity, can be difficult [38]. Both conditions share a symptom complex with abdominal pain and altered bowel habits. Moreover, IBS-like symptoms are frequently reported before the diagnosis of IBD [38, 39]. Another concern is microscopic colitis (MC). MC and IBS have similar symptoms and normal endoscopic appearance [40-47]. Diagnostic overlap between IBS and IBD on one hand, and IBS and MC in the other is important because of a potentially different treatment for each disorder. The prevalence of IBD in patients that fulfilled Rome criteria without alarming symptoms varies between 0.4 and 1.9% [46-51] and MC from 0.7 to 1.5% [41-47]. It is conceivable to conclude that symptom-based diagnosis of IBS may lead to missing a number of other gastrointestinal disorders that require quite different management to IBS. Sigmoidoscopy in IBS patients might be insufficient as a considerable number of MC may not be identified without mucosal biopsies from the right colon [46]. Furthermore, performing sigmoidoscopy would not exclude Crohn's disease lesions in the terminal ileum. Other blood tests seem to have a rather low sensitivity [38]. Ileocolonoscopy is, therefore, preferred, especially in IBS-D patients.

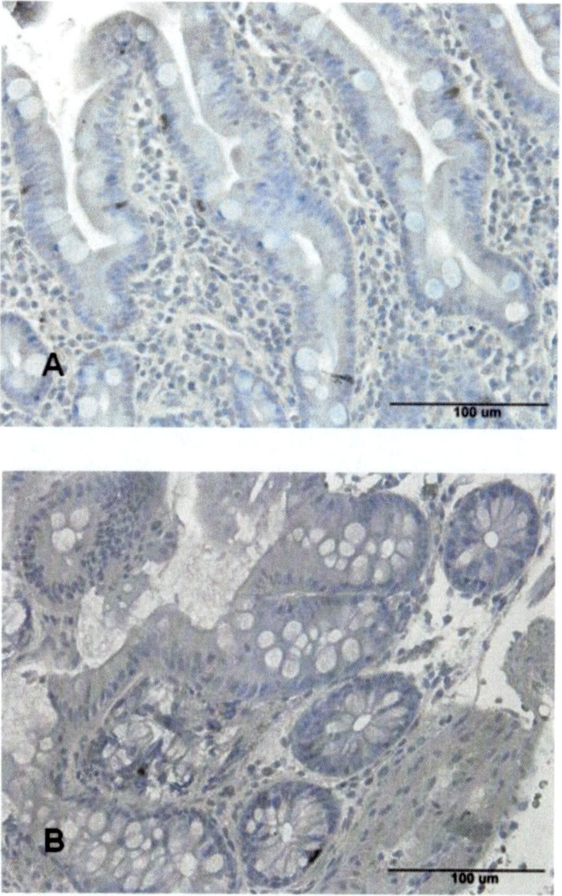

Reproduced from 59.

Figure 5. Chromogranin A positive cells in the duodenum of a healthy subject (A) and of a patient with IBS (B).

To perform ileocolonoscopy with mucosal biopsies in IBS patients seems, at first sight, as adding more economic burden to health-care, which is already suffering from a lack of resources. It also seems that resources from seriously ill patients would have to be drawn to meet this task. IBS patients are already consuming a lot of health-care resources (see Chapter 2). In fact, most IBS patients have undergone colonoscopy once or several times. Unfortunately, the doctors that refer them and those who perform colonoscopy directly or indirectly act as if they expect no pathological findings and that the examination is unnecessary. This does not reassure IBS patients and they repeatedly seek a new examination. To perform ileocolonoscopy would reassure IBS patients and prevent them from seeking a new examination. In conclusion, performing ileocolonoscopy with mucosal biopsies in IBS patients would not increase the economic burden of this patient group on society, but instead use the existing resources effectively.

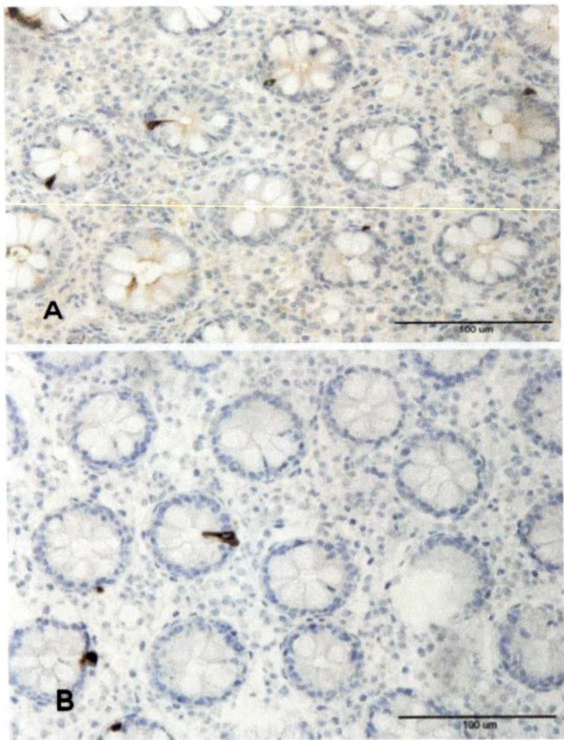

Reproduced from 59.

Figure 6. Chromogranin A immunoreactive cells in the colon of a healthy subject (A) and of a patient with IBS (B).

A wide range of biomarkers for the diagnosis of IBS have been considered, but only gut transit measured by radio-isotope markers meet the criteria for reproducibility and availability [52]. However radio-isotope tests are expensive and of limited availability [52].

We have reported that chromogranin A-containing cell density is low in the duodenum and colon of both IBS-constipation and IBS-diarrhoea patients (Figures 5, 6, & 7) [53].

As chromogranin A is a general marker for endocrine cells [54-55], this finding indicates that a general reduction in small intestinal and large intestinal endocrine cells does occur in these patients.

We have proposed that the quantification of chromogranin A cell density could be used as a histopathological marker for the diagnosis of IBS [53, 57]. Receiver-operator characteristic (ROC) curves for chromogranin A cell density in the duodenum and colon are given in Figure 8.

The sensitivity and specificity at the cut off < 31 cells/mm^2 in the duodenum are 91 and 89%. In the colon the corresponding figures with a cut off <30 cells/mm^2 are 81 sensitivity and 88% specificity. It is worth noting that these results are based on 41 patients and 42 controls for the duodenum and 41 patients and 17 controls in the colon.

These results demonstrate that chromogranin A cell density has a higher sensitivity and specificity in the duodenal tissue than in colon specimens. This may be due to the fact that the duodenum harbours almost all the endocrine cell types expressed by the small intestine and in a large number [58]. Furthermore, it is much easier and more acceptable for the patients if duodenal biopsies are obtained by gastroscopy, rather than obtaining colon biopsies using colonoscopy.

As duodenal biopsies provide more sensitive and specific results, and this method would be preferred over the collection analysis of colonic biopsies to determine chromogranin A cell density. Screening of IBS patients for celiac disease is now widely accepted.

Thus, gastroscopy with duodenal biopsies can be used for excluding or confirming celiac disease instead of blood tests and the same biopsies can be used for the diagnosis of IBS.

The rectum comprises a larger number of endocrine cells than the colon and is probably more suitable to be used in diagnosis. The results in our laboratory showed, unfortunately, that chromogranin A cell density in the rectum of IBS patients does not differ from that of controls (unpublished data).

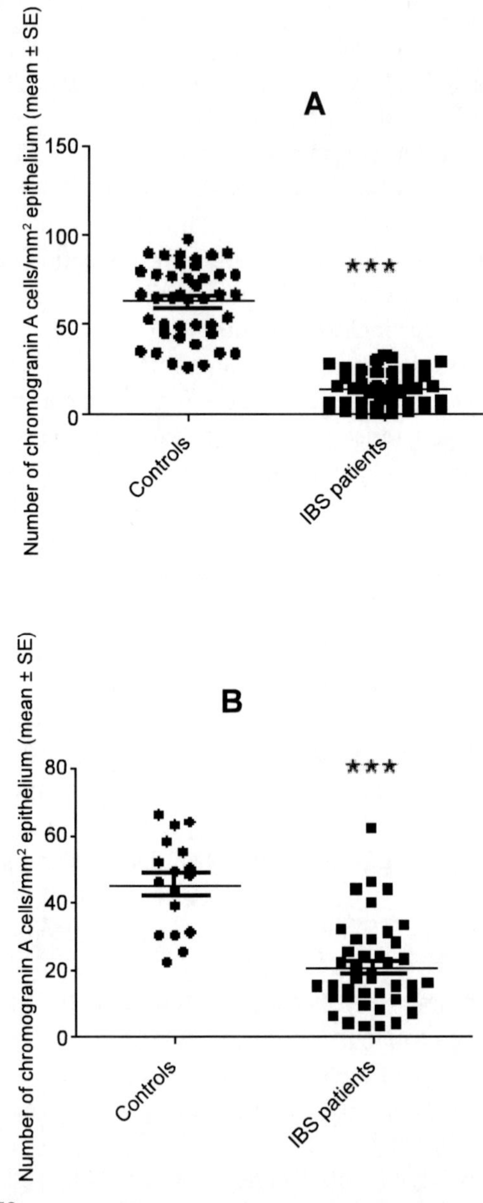

Reproduced from 59.

Figure 7. Chromogranin A cell density in the duodenum (A) and in the colon (B) of controls and IBS patients.

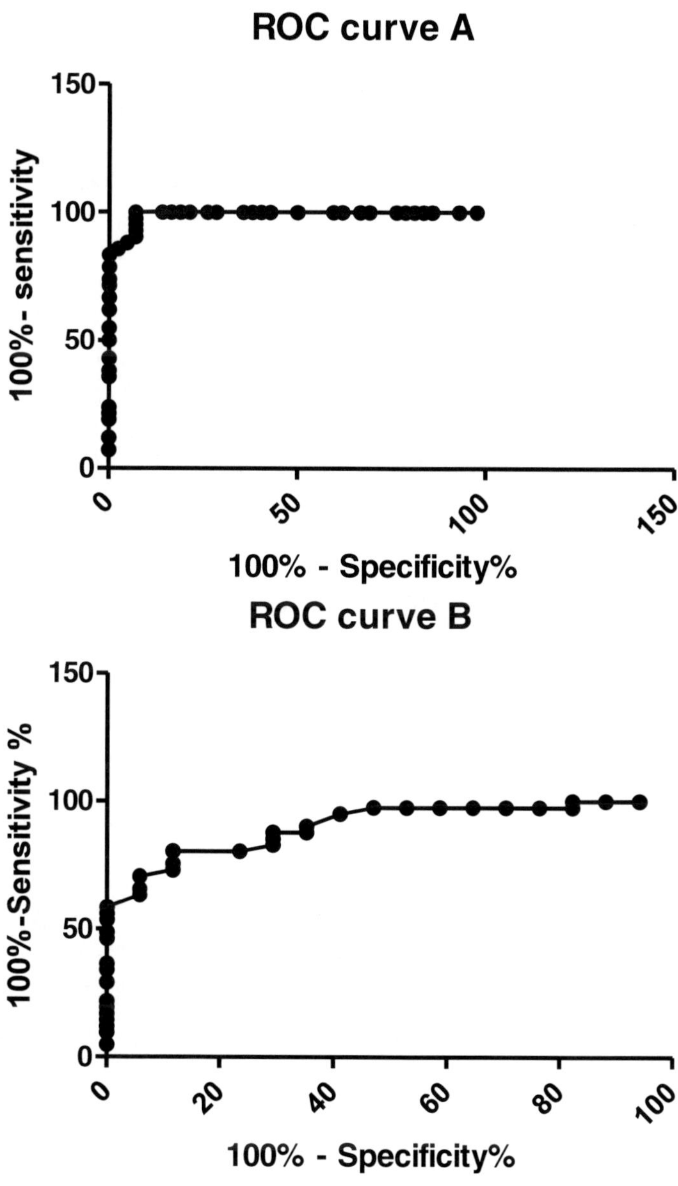

Figure 8. Receiver-operator characteristic (ROC) for chromogranin A cell density in the duodenum (A) and in the colon (B). Reproduced from 59.

References

[1]   Manning AP, Thompson WG, Heaton KW, Morris AF. Towards positive diagnosis of the irritable bowel. *Br Med J.* 1978; 2: 653-654.

[2]   Drossman DA, Thompson WG, Talley NJ, et al. Identification of subgroups of functional gastrointestinal disorders. *Gastroenterol Int* 1990; 3: 159-172.

[3]   Thompson WG, Longstreth GF, Drossman DA, Heaton KW, Irvine EJ, Müller-Lissner SA. Functional bowel disorders and functional abdominal pain. *Gut* 1999; 45 (Suppl 2): II43-II47.

[4]   Longstreth GF, Thompson WG, Chey WD, Valenzuela-Barranco M, Martín-Ruiz JL, Herrerías-Gutiérrez JM, Esteban-Carretero JM. Functional bowel disorders. *Gastroenterology* 260; 130: 1480-1491.

[5]   Mearin F, Balboa A, Badía X, Baró E, Caldwell E, Cucala M, Díaz-Rubio M, Fueyo A, Ponce J, Roset M, Talley NJ. Irritable bowel syndrome subtypes according to bowel habit: revisiting the alternating subtype. *Eur J Gastroenterol Hepatol.* 2003; 15: 165-172.

[6]   Tillisch K, Labus JS, Naliboff BD, Bolus R, Shetzline M, Mayer EA, Chang L. Characterization of the alternating bowel habit subtype in patients with irritable bowel syndrome. *Am J Gastroenterol.* 2005;100: 896-904.

[7]   Drossman DA, Morris CB, Hu Y, Toner BB, Diamant N, Leserman J, Shetzline, M, Dalton, C, Bangdiwala SI. A prospective assessment of bowel habit in irritable bowel syndrome in women: defining an alternator. *Gastroenterology* 2005; 128: 580-589.

[8]   Whitehead WE, Drossman DA.Validation of symptom-based diagnostic criteria for irritable bowel syndrome: a critical review. *Am J Gastroenterol* 2010; 105: 814-820.

[9]   Lea R, Hopkins V, Hastleton J, Houghton LA, Whorwell PJ. Diagnostic criteria for irritable bowel syndrome: utility and applicability in clinical practice. *Digestion* 2004; 70: 210-213.

[10]   Gladman LM, Gorard DA. General practitioner and hospital specialist attitudes to functional gastrointestinal disorders. *Aliment Pharmacol Ther* 2003; 17: 651–654.

[11]   Thompson WG, Heaton KW, Smyth GT, Smyth C. Irritable bowel syndrome in general practice: Prevalence, characteristics, and referral. *Gut* 2000; 46: 78–82.

[12] Corsetti M, Tack. Are symptom-based diagnostic criteria for irritable bowel syndrome useful in clinical practice? *Digestion* 2004; 70: 207-209.

[13] Whitehead EW, Palsson OS, Feld AD, Levy RL, Von Korff M, Turner MJ, Drossman DA. Utility of red flag symptom exclusions in the diagnosis of irritable bowel syndrome. *Almiment Pharmacol ther* 2006; 24: 137-146.

[14] American College of Gastroenterology Task Force on Irritable Bowel Syndrome: An evidence-based position statement on the management of irritable bowel syndrome. *Am J Gastroenterol* 2009; 104: S1-35.

[15] Spiller R, Aziz Q, Creed F, Emmanuel A, Houghton L, Hungin P, Jones R, Kumor D, Rubin G, Trudgill N, Whorwell P. Guidelines on the irritable bowel syndrome: mechanisms and practical management. *Gut* 2007; 56: 1770-1798.

[16] Sanders DS, Carter MJ, Hurlstone DP, Pearce A, Ward AM, MCAlindon ME, Lobo AJ. Association of adult celiac disease with irritable bowel syndrome: a case-control study in patients fulfilling Rome criteria referred to secondary care. *Lancet* 2001; 358: 1504-1508.

[17] Ziper RD, Patel S, Yahya KZ, BaischDW, Monarch E. Presentation of adult celiac disease in nationwide patient support group. *Dig Dis Sci* 2003; 48: 761-764.

[18] Wahnscaffe U, Ulrch R, Reiken EO, Sculzke JD. Celiac disease-like abnormalities in subgroup of patients with irritable bowel syndrome. *Gastroenterolgy* 2001; 121: 1329-1338.

[19] Bottaro G, Calado F, Rotolo N, Spina M, Corazza GR. The clinical pattern of subclinical/silent celiac disease: an analysis on 1026-consecutive cases. *Am J Gastroenterol* 1999; 94:691-696.

[20] Green PHR, Stavropoulos SN, Panagi SG, Goldstein SL, McMahon DJ, Absan H, Neugut AI. Characteristics of adult celiac disease in USA: results of a national survey. *Am J Gastroenterol* 2001; 96: 126-131.

[21] Lo W, Sano K, Lebwohl B, Diamond B, Green PH. Changing presentation of adult celiac disease. *Dig Dis Sci* 2003; 48: 395-298.

[22] El-Salhy M, Lomholt-Beck B, Gundersen D. The prevalence of celiac disease in patients with irritable bowel syndrome. *Mol Med Rep* 2011; 4: 403-405.

[23] Eswaran S, Tack J, Chey WD. Food: the forgotten factor in the irritable bowel syndrome. *Gastro Clin N Amr* 2011; 40: 141-162.

[24] Fasano A, Berti I, Geraduzzi D, Not T, Colletti RB, Drago S, Elitsur Y, Green PH, Guandalini S, Hill ID, Pietzak M, Ventura A, Thorpe M,

Kryszak D, Fornaroli F, Wasserman SS, Murray JA, Horvath K. Prevalence of celiac disease in at-risk and not-at-risk groups in USA: a large multicentre study. *Arch Intern Med* 2003; 163: 286-292.

[25] Wouden E, Nelis JF, Vecht J. Screening for coeliac disease in patients fulfilling Rome II criteria for irritable bowel syndrome in a secondary care hospital in The Netherlands: a prospective observational study. *Gut* 2007; 56: 444-445.

[26] Locke GR 3rd, Murry JA, Zinsmeister A, Melton LJ 3rd, Talley NJ. Celiac disease serology in irritable bowel syndrome and dyspepsia: a population based case-control study. *Mayo Clin Proc* 2004; 79: 476-482.

[27] Hin H, Bird G, Fisher P, Mahy N, Jewell D. Celiac disease in primary care: case finding study. *BMJ* 1999; 318: 164-167.

[28] Shahbazhkhani B, Forootan M, Merat S, Akbari MR, Nasserimoghadam S, Vahedi H, Malekzadeh R. Celiac disease presenting with symptoms of irritable bowel syndrome. *Aliment Pharmacol Ther* 2003; 18: 231-235.

[29] Catassi C, Kryzak D, Louis-Jacques O, Duerksen DR, Hill I, Crowe SE, Brown AR, Procaccini NJ, Wonderly BA, Hartley P, Moreci J, Bennett N, Horvath K, Burk M, Fasano A. Detection of celiac disease in primary care: a multicenter case-finding study in North America. *Am J Gastroenterol* 2007; 102: 1454-1460.

[30] Korkut E, Bektas M, Oztas E, Kurt M, Cetinkaya H, Ozden A. The prevalence o f celiac disease in patients fulfilling Rome III criteria for irritable bowel syndrome. *Eur J Intern Med* 2010; 21: 389-392.

[31] Sanders DS, Patel D, Stephenson TJ, Ward AM, McCloskey EV, Hadjivassiliou M, Lobo AJ. A primary care cross-sectional study of undiagnosed adult coeliac disease. *Eur J Gastroenterol Hepatol* 2003; 15: 407-413.

[32] Holt R, Darnley S, Kennedy T, Jones R. Screening for coeliac disease in patients with clinical diagnosis of irritable bowel syndrome. *Gastroenterology* 2001; 120: A757-A808.

[33] Verdu EF, Armstrong D, Murry JA. Between celiac disease and irritable bowel syndrome: the "no man's land" of gluten sensitivity. *Am J Gastroenterol* 2009; 104: 1587-1594.

[34] Wahnschaffe U, Schulzke JD, Zeitz M, Ullrich R. Predictors of clinical response to gluten free diet in patients diagnosed with diarrhea-predominant irritable bowel syndrome. *Clin Gastroenterol Hepatol* 2007; 5: 844-850.

[35] Monsbakken KW, Vandvik PO, Farup PG. Perceived food intolerance in subjects with irritable bowel syndrome-etiology, prevalence and consequences. *Eur J Clin Nutr* 2005; 60: 667-672.

[36] Young E, Stoneham MD, Petruckevitc A, Barton J, Rona R. A population study of food intolerance. *Lancet* 1994; 343: 1127-1130.

[37] Schoepfer AM, Trummler M, Seeholzer P, Schoepfer AM, Trummler M, Seeholzer P, Seibold-Schmid B, Seibold F. Discriminating IBD from IBS: comparison of the test performance of fecal markers, blood leukocytes, CRP and IBD antibodies. *Inflamm Bowel Dis* 2008; 14: 32-39.

[38] Bercik P, Verdu EF, Collins SM. Is irritable bowel syndrome a low-grade inflammatory bowel disease? *Gastroenterol Clin North Am* 2005; 34: 235-245.

[39] Burgman T, Clara I, Graff L, Walker J, Lix L, Rawsthorne P, McPhail C, Rogala L, Miller N, Bernstein CN. The Manitoba inflammatory bowel disease. Cohort study: prolonged symptoms before diagnosis-how much is irritable bowel syndrome? *Clin Gastroenterol Hepatol* 2006; 4: 614-620.

[40] Drossman DA, Camilleri M, Mayer EA, Whitehead WE. AGA technical review on irritable bowel syndrome. *Gastroenterology* 2002; 123: 2108-2131.

[41] Limsui D, Pardi DS, Camilleri M, Loftus EV Jr, Kammer PP, Tremaine WJ, Sandborn WJ. Symptomatic overlap between irritable bowel syndrome and microscopic colitis. *Inflamm Bowel Dis* 2007; 13: 175-181.

[42] Barta Z, Mekkel G, Csipo I, Tóth L, Szakáll S, Szabó GG, Bakó G, Szegedi G, Zeher M. Microscopic colitis: a retrospective study of clinical presentation in 53 patients. *World J Gastroenterol* 2005; 11: 1351-1355.

[43] Madisch A, Bethke B, Stolte M, Miehlke S. Is there an association of microscopic colitis and irritable bowel syndrome -a subgroup analysis of placebo-controlled trial. *World J Gastroenterol* 2005; 11: 6409.

[44] Kao KT, Pedraza BA, McClune AC, Rios DA, Mao YQ, Zuch RH, Kanter MH, Wirio S, Conteas CN. Microscopic colitis: a large retrospective analysis from health maintenance organization experience. *World J Gastroenterol* 2009; 15: 3122-3127.

[45] Yantiss R, Odze R. Optimal approach to obtain mucosal biopsies for assessment of inflammatory disorders of the gastrointestinal tract. *Am J Gastroenterol* 2009; 104: 774-783.

[46] Fissora Cl, Koch KL. Symptom overlap and comorbidity of irritable bowel syndrome with other conditions. *Curr Gastroenterol Rep* 2005; 7: 264-271.

[47] El-Salhy M, Halwe J, Lomholt-Beck B, Gundersen D. The prevalence of inflammatory bowel diseases, microscopic colitis and colorectal cancer in patients with irritable bowel syndrome. *Gastroenterol Insights* 2011; 3: 7-10.

[48] Tolliver BA,Herrera JL, DiPalma JA. Evaluation of patients who meet clinical criteria for irritable bowel syndrome. *Am J Gastroenterol* 1994; 89: 176-178.

[49] Hamm LR, Sorrells SC, Harding JP, Northcutt AR, Heath AT, Kapke GF, Hunt CM, Mangel AW. Additional investigations fail to alter the diagnosis of irritable bowel syndrome in subjects fulfilling the Rome criteria. *Am J Gstroenterol* 1999; 94: 1279-1282.

[50] Vanner SJ, Depew WT, Paterson WG, DaCosta LR, Groll AG, Simon JB, Djurfeldt. Predictive values of the Rome criteria for diagnosing the irritable bowel syndrome. *Am J Gastroenterol* 1999; 94: 2912-2917.

[51] MacIntosh DG, Thompson WG, Patel DG, Barr R, Guindi M. Is rectal biopsy necessary in irritable bowel syndrome? *Am J Gastroenterol* 1992; 87: 1407-1409.

[52] Spiller RC. Potential biomarkers. *Gastroenterol Clin North Am* 2011; 40: 121-139.

[53] El-Salhy M, Lomholt-Beck B, Hausken T. Chromogranin as a tool in the diagnosis of irritable bowel syndrome. *Scan J Gastroenterol* 2010; 45: 1435-1439.

[54] Taupenot L, Harper KL, O`Connor DT. The chromogranin-secretogranin family. *N Engl J Med* 2003; 348: 1134-1149.

[55] Wicdenmann B, Huttner WB. Synaptophysin and Chromogranin /secretogranins-widespread constituents of distinct types of neuroendocrine vesicles and new tools in tumor diagnosis. *Virchows Arch B Cell Pathol* 1989; 58: 95-121.

[56] Deftos LJ. Chromogranin A: its role in endocrine function and as an endocrine and neuroendocrine tumor marker. *Endocrine Reviews* 1991; 12:181-188.

[57] El-Salhy M, Seim I, Chopin L, Gundersen D, Hatlebakk JG, Hausken T. Irritable bowel syndrome: the role of gut neuroendocrine peptides. *Front Biosci* 2012; E4: 2683-2700.

[58] Sandström O, El-Salhy M. Aging and endocrine cells of human duodenum. *Mech. Ageing Develop.* 1999; 108: 39-48.

Chapter IV

Pathogenesis of Irritable Bowel Syndrome

Abstract

The pathogenesis of IBS seems to be multifactorial, where several factors have been suggested to play a role in this process such as psychological factors, genetic factors, an abnormal neuroendocrine system (NES) in the gut and/or altered signalling in this system, dietary factors, intestinal flora and low-grade chronic intestinal inflammation. There is evidence to show that the following factors play a central role in the pathogenesis of IBS: hereditability and genetic, dietary/intestinal microbiota, low-grade inflammation and disturbed NES of the gut. We have proposed the following hypothesis: the cause of IBS is an altered NES. An altered NES would cause abnormal gastrointestinal motility, secretion and sensation. All of these abnormalities are characteristic of IBS. The alteration in NES could be a result of one or more of the following: genetic factors, dietary intake, intestinal flora or low-grade inflammation. In support of this hypothesis: 1. abnormalities have been reported in the neuroendocrine peptides/amines of the gut. These abnormalities would cause disturbances in digestion, gastrointestinal motility and visceral hypersensitivity. 2. The genetic difference between IBS patients and healthy subjects was found in the genes controlling the serotonin signalling system and cholecystokinin (CCK). 3. The differences in diet, intestinal flora and inflammation affect the NES of the gut. The release of different gut hormones depends of the composition and quantity of the food ingested. The food content of FODMAPs (fermentable oligosaccharides, disaccharides, monosaccharides and polyols) and fibres, and intestinal flora and subsequent fermentation, increase the osmotic pressure in the intestines. This change in intestinal pressure stimulates the release of hormones such as serotonin. Likewise, inflammation and the release of secretory products from immune cells affect the release of hormones and the proliferation of gut endocrine cells.

The pathogenesis of IBS appears to be multifactorial and several aspects have been suggested to play a role in this process. Thus, psychological factors, genetic factors, an abnormal neuroendocrine system in the gut and/or altered signalling in this system, dietary factors, intestinal flora and low-grade chronic intestinal inflammation are discussed.

4.1. Psychological Factors

Irritable bowel syndrome is a chronic disorder and one would expect that IBS patients have the same distress as other patients with chronic diseases such as inflammatory bowel diseases (IBD) patients. Whereas IBD patients receive effective treatment and are treated with sympathy, understanding and support by their doctors as well as society, IBS patients are offered non-effective treatments, are treated with mistrust and neglect by their doctors and feel that they are labelled as hypochondriacs and receive no support from society. One would expect that, as a normal reaction, these patients would be more anxious and depressed than IBD patients. However, one should be careful not to mix effect and cause.

In an epidemiological study on patients diagnosed with IBS among the adult residents of Olmsted County, Minnesota, USA, 2% were found to suffer from depression [1]. The incidence of depression in these patients was low compared to the incidence of depression found for the entire population of the United States, which was 16.2% [2]. A prospective multicenter study on a supposedly representative sample (208 patients) of patients with IBS in a Norwegian general practice showed that the IBS patients had an increased prevalence of depression compared to the background population [3], where the prevalence of depression in IBS patients was 37% and in normal subjects (1240 subjects) it was 2.7%. The prevalence of depression in the normal subjects used in this study is incredibly low compared to worldwide estimates of the prevalence of depression. In the study they referred to as the source for the control subjects, 65% of these subjects reported pseudoneurological complaints such as tiredness, depression and dizziness [4]. Furthermore, in another study performed on a random sample (2066 subjects) of the adult population of Oslo, the prevalence of depression has been found to be 17.8% [5].

Several studies have shown that a large proportion of IBS patients suffer from depression, anxiety, hypochondriasis and somatisation [6-10]. In a review of the comorbidity of IBS with other disorders, psychiatric disorders, especially depression, anxiety and somatoform disorders were found to occur in up to 94% of patients [11]. In order to establish whether or not psychiatric disorders occur before or after the onset of IBS symptoms, 188 treatment-seeking IBS patients were examined [6] and it was found that anxiety is the most likely disorder to develop before the onset of IBS symptoms [6].

It has been argued that the effectiveness of antidepressants and the response to anxiolytic treatment, as well as psychological treatment, support the notion that a psychological component is important in IBS symptomology in some patients [12]. About 95% of serotonin in the body is expressed in the gastrointestinal tract and is synthesised by enterochromaffin (EC) cells and sertonergic neurons of the myenteric plexus [13]. Antidepressant and anxiolytic drugs increase the concentration of serotonin at its receptors by inhibiting its uptake. Is it possible that the effects exerted by these drugs on IBS patients are due to their effects at the gut rather than on the central nervous system? Moreover, are psychological consults of other patients with chronic gastrointestinal disease less beneficial?

Several reports have shown an association between sexual and physical abuse and IBS [14-21]. It has been postulated that abuse could induce the expression of neuroticism, which in turn leads to IBS [21]. On the other hand, it has been reported that rectal hypersensitivity and poor health status in IBS patients are not related to sexual and/or physical abuse [22,23].

Twenty-five years ago, Creed and Guthrie [24] wrote "The role of psychological factors in the aetiology of the IBS is far from clear, but a review of the literature suggests that some consistent patterns are emerging in spite of methodological problems. There have been three major defects with studies that have linked IBS with neurotic symptomatology. First, the measurement of psychological factors has generally been imprecise. Second, most studies have considered IBS patients as a single group, without making allowance for differing symptom patterns. Third, conclusions have been drawn about hospital samples and extrapolated to IBS subjects, without taking account of factors which affect consulting behaviour" Twenty years later, Spiller and colleagues stated that. "The role of psychological factors in the onset and progress of IBS is complex, and remains controversial" [12]. One wonders whether this statement can still be true today.

4.2. Hereditability and Environmental and Social Learning

Evidence for hereditability as a factor in the aetiology of IBS is based on clinical observations of family clustering, familial aggregation investigations and twin and genetic studies [25].

4.2.1. Familial Aggregation

Family clustering of IBS was noticed several years ago in clinical practice. The familial aggregation of IBS has been confirmed by several studies [26-29]. Whorwell and co-workers found that 33% of patients with IBS had a family history of IBS compared to 2% of the controls [26].

A significant association between having a first degree family member with bowel symptoms and presenting with IBS was shown in a study of a family cluster of 643 subjects from Olmsted County, USA. Those who reported having a spouse with bowel symptoms were not more likely to present with IBS [27].

In another study [28], it was shown that the prevalence of IBS was 17% in patients' relatives compared to 7% in the relatives of spouses. Another study showed that patients with IBS were more likely than controls to present a family history of IBS (33.9% vs. 12.6%). Moreover, of IBS non-consulter patients, 21.1% reported a family history of IBS compared to 12.6% of the controls [29].

4.2.2. Twin Studies

In an Australian study of 343 twin pairs, a higher rate of IBS was reported in monozygotic twins than in dizygotic twins (33.3% vs. 13.3%). Moreover, 56.9% of the variance was attributed to additive genetic factors, indicating a substantial genetic component in IBS [30].

Two twin studies on IBS were conducted in the USA. The first study included 6060 twin pairs from the Commonwealth of Virginia, USA. This study showed that the rate of IBS was significantly greater in monozygotic twins (17.2) than in dizygotic twins (8.4), supporting a genetic contribution to IBS [31]. The second study included 986 twin pairs randomly selected from the Minnesota Twin Registry, USA.

The polychoric correlation for monozygotic twins with IBS (47%) was substantially larger than that for dizygotic twins (17%). Genetic modelling has confirmed the independent additive genetic effect in IBS. Adjusting for anxiety and depression reduced the difference so that no statistical significance remained. The authors concluded that there is a genetic contribution to IBS that could be mediated by hereditability for anxiety and depression [32]. However, an American study performed on 288 Swedish twin pairs showed that there are no genetic or familial environmental factors that explain the association between major depressive diseases and IBS [33].

Norwegian twin pairs identified from the Norwegian national registry (3286 twin pairs) were investigated for IBS. This study has showed that the rate of IBS was significantly greater in monozygotic twins (22.4%) than in dizygotic twins (9.1%).

Furthermore, the heritability of IBS was estimated to be 48.4% among females [34]. In contrast to the twins studies presented above, a twins study performed on 1870 British twin pairs did not show any significance in the rates of IBS between monozygotic and dizygotic twins [35].

4.2.3. Genetic Studies

The serotonin transporter (SERT) gene encoding the SERT protein is located on chromosome 17q11.2-q1. A functional polymorphism is an insertion or a deletion of 44 base pairs in the SERT-gene-linked polymorphic region (5-HTTLPR) [25].

An association was reported between a functional polymorphism in the serotonin transporter (SERT) gene and diarrhoea-predominant IBS [36,37].

Individuals with a long allele genotype of the SERT gene have been shown to be vulnerable to developing IBS with constipation [38], and a polymorphism in the cholecystokinin([CCK) CCKAR gene (779T>C) has also been found to be associated with IBS with constipation [39].

4.2.4. Environment and Social Learning

Several studies have shown that parental modelling and the reinforcement of illness behaviour can contribute to the causes of IBS [40-44]. It has been reported that having a mother with IBS accounts for as much variance as having an identical set of genes with a co-twin who has IBS, suggesting that the contribution of social learning to IBS is at least as great as the contribution of heredity [40]. The authors showed this was not due to a halo effect, i.e., a tendency to attribute the symptoms one has to others because one has become sensitised to noticing them [40].

4.3. Dietary Factors

Patients with IBS believe that their diet has a significant influence on their symptoms and they are interested in finding out which foods they should avoid [45-48].

4.3.1. Diet Intake in IBS Patients

About 60% of IBS patients report a worsening of symptoms following food ingestion: 28% within 15 minutes after eating and 93% within 3 hours [49]. Many IBS patients report specific foods, most commonly implicating milk and milk products, wheat products, onion, peas/beans, hot spices, cabbage, certain meats, smoked products, fried food and caffeine as the offending foods [49,50]. Therefore, one would expect that IBS patients would be selective in their choice of food. However, dietary surveys among IBS patients in the community failed to detect any differences in dietary composition between IBS patients and community controls [51-54] (Figures 9 and 10). However, a Norwegian study on food intolerance and IBS showed that 62% of the subjects had limited or excluded food items from their daily intake and that 12% of these had made changes to their diet that were so drastic that nutritional deficiencies could be possible in the long run [55]. In a recent study, IBS patients were reported to have made a conscious choice to avoid certain food items, some of which belong to FODMAPs (fermentable oligosaccharides, disaccharides, monosaccharides and polyols). However, they reported a higher consumption of other food items that are rich in FODMAPs [54].They also reportedly avoided other food sources that are important for health. Furthermore, IBS patients have also been reported to have a lower alcohol consumption [49,54-56] and intolerance to various alcoholic beverages, and as many as 12% either limit or avoid such beverages [49,54].

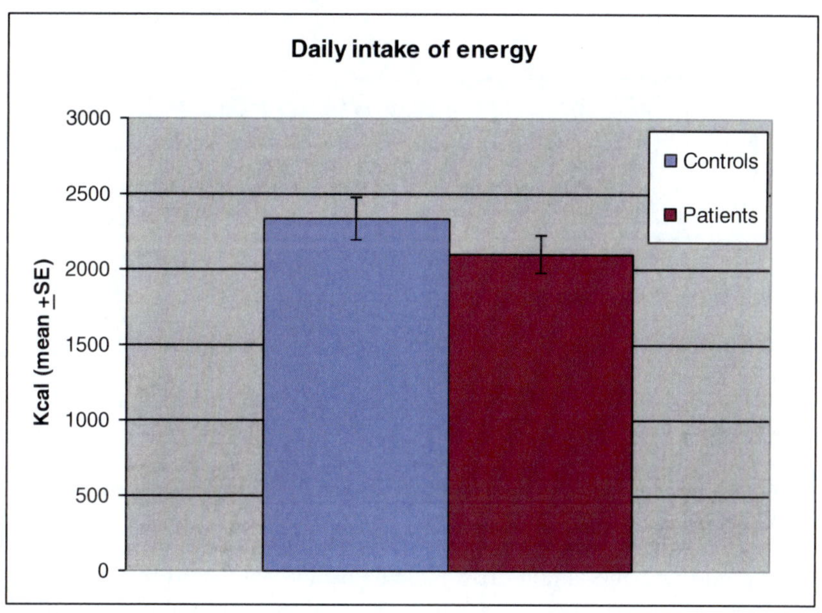

Data from 54.

Figure 9. No significant difference was found in the daily energy intake between healthy subjects and IBS patients.

Irritable bowel syndrome patients have reported a lower consumption of spaghetti, pasta, rice, millet, couscous and buns than controls. Spaghetti, pasta and couscous are products made from durum wheat, which tends to be high in FODMAPs, whereas rice tends to be low in FODMAPs [54,55-57]. Furthermore, IBS patients reported a lower consumption of certain vegetables (raw vegetables, raw broccoli, paprika, onion, leeks, garlic, cabbage, tomatoes, mushrooms and green beans) [54].This is the most likely reason for the significantly lower intake of retinol equivalents, beta-carotene and magnesium observed in these patients [54] (Figure 12). On the other hand, IBS patients have reported a higher level of consumption of grapes, pears, peach, beans, mango, plums and melon [54].These are all fruits and vegetables that are rich in FODMAPs and that have been reported to be causal factors of symptoms.

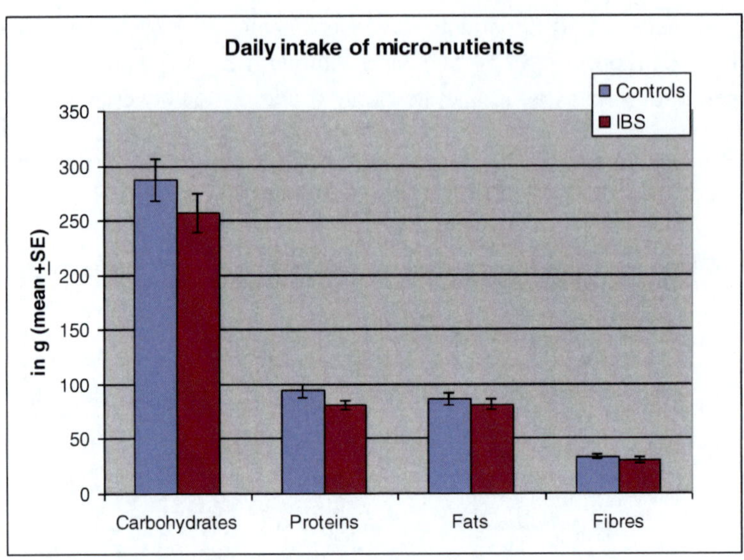

Data from 54.

Figure 10. Both healthy subjects and IBS patients were found to have a similar daily intake of macronutrients.

The common belief among IBS patients is that lactose is the main cause of their symptoms [57]. They have reported a lower consumption of milk and milk products (Figure 11) [54]. Milk and other dairy products are the most important dietary source of calcium, vitamin B2 [riboflavin] and phosphorus in the Western world, and the calcium, vitamin B2 and phosphorus content of these food items can contribute up to 50-75%, 30% and 20-30%, respectively, of the daily dietary intake of these nutrients [49,55,57]. However, IBS patients also reported a much higher consumption of alternative milk products such as soy, rice and oat milk [56], although IBS patients still have a low intake of calcium, vitamin B2 and phosphorus (Figure 12) [54].

4.3.2. Food Allergy/Intolerance in IBS Patients?

Food allergy or intolerance has been thought to be the cause of IBS problems with certain food items. However, food allergies exist in 6-8% of children and 1-4% of adults [59].The term "food allergy" is used when a clear allergic response to a specific food item has been identified, such as a response to peanuts and fish. Characteristically, the food allergy reaction occurs rapidly and manifests as swelling, itching, hives, wheezing, nausea, vomiting, diarrhoea, abdominal pain, and/or collapse usually within less than 2 hours after ingesting the offending food item. This reaction is mediated by immunoglobulin E (IgE). There is no consistent evidence to show a role of this type of allergic response in IBS [60-65]. A slow-onset food allergy can be mediated by mucosal mechanisms in IBS; these mucosal mechanisms involve IgE, T lymphocytes, eosinophils, mast cells and other mucosal cells. The symptoms caused by this reaction develop days after the ingestion of the offending food, as supported by reports of an abnormal increase in mucosal eosinophils and mast cells in IBS [66,67].

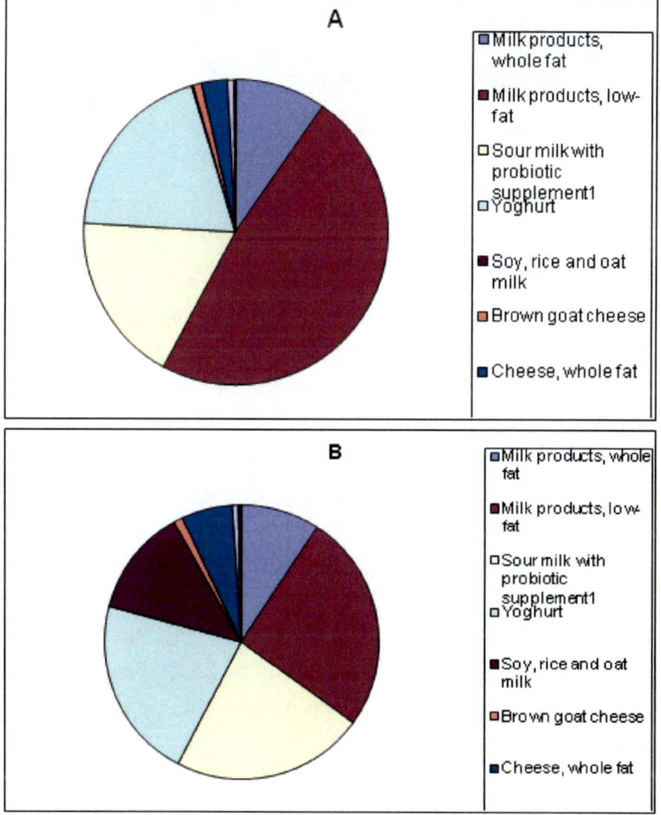

Data from 54.

Figure 11. Daily intake of dairy products by healthy subjects (A) and IBS patients (B).

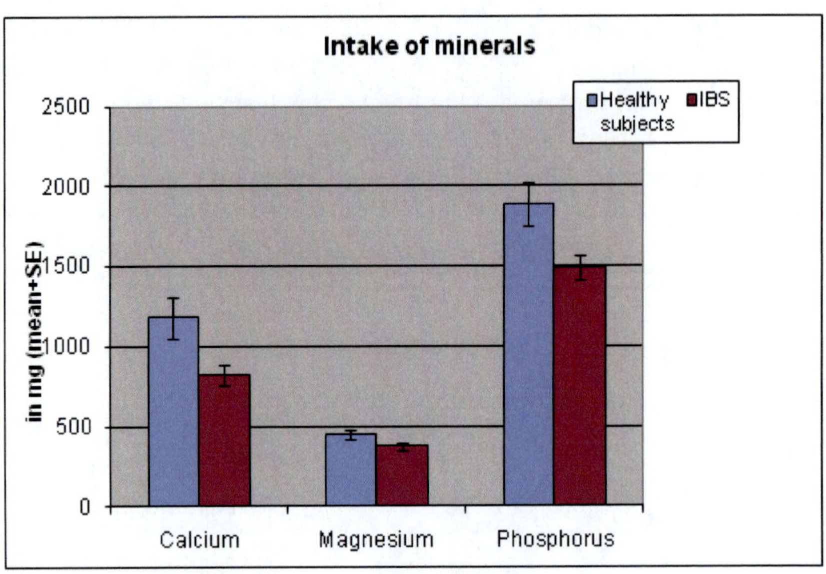

Data from 54.*=P<0.05.

Figure 12. The daily intake of vitamins and minerals was found to differ between healthy subjects and IBS patients [54].

However, these mechanisms might only be the cause of IBS symptoms in a subset of patients, some of whom also have atopy [68 ,69]. A new concept is that a different antibody class (IgG) might be implicated in food-related allergies in IBS [70-72].

However, this concept is unclear and controversial [66, 73-75]; the tests that were undertaken to support this concept are not sensitive or specific enough for clinical use [65, 71, 75-81].

About 20-70% of IBS patients complain of subjective food intolerances [49, 65, 82-88].

Food intolerances are non-toxic, non-immune-mediated adverse reactions to food, including pharmacological reactions to bioactive chemicals in foods such as histamines, sulphites, monosodium glutamate, serotonin, norepinepherine and tyramine.

Furthermore, food intolerance has a wide spectrum of symptoms, but these symptoms usually manifest outside the gastrointestinal tract in the form of headache, asthma and urticaria. There is no documented evidence showing that food intolerance plays a role in IBS symptoms.

4.3.3. Fermentable Oligo-, Di- and Monosaccharides and Polyols

The reaction of IBS patients to certain food items has recently been attributed to a number of short-chain carbohydrates that are poorly absorbed so that a significant portion of the ingested carbohydrates enters the distal small bowel and colon. Once there they increase the osmotic pressure and provide a substrate for bacterial fermentation. This in turn results in the production of gas, distension of the large intestine and abdominal discomfort or pain. These carbohydrates are fermentable oligo-, di-and monosaccharides and polyols (FODMAPs) and include fructose, lactose, sugar alcohols (sorbitol, maltitol, mannitol, xylitol and ismalt), fructans and galactans. Fructose and lactose are present in apples, pears, watermelon, honey, fruit juices, dried fruits and milk and milk products. Polyols are used in low calorie food products. Galactans and fructans are present in common dietary constituents such as wheat, rye, garlic, onions, legumes, cabbage, artichokes, leeks, asparagus, lentils, inulin, soy, Brussels sprouts and broccoli [47,48].

4.3.4. Dietary Fibre

A deficiency in dietary fibre was widely believed to be the primary cause of IBS (89). Although increasing the amount of dietary fibre continues to be a standard recommendation for patients with IBS, clinical practice has shown that increased fibre intake in these patients increases abdominal pain, bloating and distension. An evaluation of the efficacy of fibre as a treatment for IBS was the subject of a recent review and meta-analysis that included 12 trials. This review shows that patients assigned to the fibre treatment showed persistent symptoms or no improvement in symptoms after treatment compared to the placebo or a low-fibre diet. Other studies have shown that whilst a water-insoluble fibre intake did not improve IBS symptoms, soluble-fibre intake was effective in improving overall IBS symptoms [90,91].

It is noteworthy that the role of FODMAPs and fibre on IBS symptoms is associated with intestinal flora. The presence of bacteria that break down FODMAPs and fibre and produce gas, such as Clostridia spp., can cause distension of the large intestine with abdominal discomfort or pain.

4.4. Intestinal Flora

Most bacteria in the gastrointestinal tract occur in the colon. The colon of each individual contains between 300 and 500 different species of bacteria [92]. Each person has their own unique intestinal flora. The intestinal flora is affected by several factors such as diet, climate changes, stress, illness, aging and antibiotic treatment [92]. The intestinal flora in IBS patients has been found to differ considerably from that of healthy controls [93]. Irritable bowel syndrome patients have fewer Lactobacillus and Bifdobacterium spp. than healthy subjects [94]. These bacteria bind to epithelial cells and inhibit pathogen binding and enhance barrier functioning [94]. Furthermore, these bacterial species do not produce gas upon fermenting carbohydrates, an effect that would be amplified as they also inhibit the Clostridia spp. [94]. Probiotics alter colonic fermentation and stabilize the colonic microbiota, and several studies on probiotics have shown improvements in flatulence and abdominal distension with a reduction in the composite IBS symptom score [94-96].

4.5. Low-Grade Inflammation

Following bacterial gastroenteritis, about 25% of patients show IBS-D type at 6 months post-infection and an average of about 10% develop persistent symptoms [97-100]. Post-infectious (PI)-IBS has been reported after Campylobacter, Salmonella and Shigella infections [97]. The incidence of PI-IBS varies between 7 to 31%, although the largest studies agreed on about 10% [97-100]. One study showed that 6 to 17% of sporadic (unselected) IBS patients believed that their symptoms began with an infection [97]. Following infection the initial inflammatory response shows an increase in CD3 lymphocytes, CD8 intraepithelial lymphocytes and calprotectin-positive macrophages [101]. These changes rapidly decrease in most subjects but a small number with persistent symptoms fail to show this decline [101]. Furthermore, the number of serotonin cells was shown to increase in these subjects with persistent symptoms [101]. There are several pieces of evidence showing that inflammation and immune cells affect the neuroendocrine system of the gut (NES), which controls and regulates gastrointestinal motility and sensitivity [102]. Thus, serotonin secretion by enterochromaffin (EC) cells can be enhanced or attenuated by secretory products of immune cells such as CD4+T [103]. Furthermore, serotonin modulates the immune response [103].

The EC are in contact with or very close to CD3+ and CD20+ lymphocytes and several serotonergic receptors have been characterised in lymphocytes, monocytes, macrophages and dendritic cells [104].Moreover, immune cells in the small and large intestine show receptors for substance P and vasoactive intestinal polypeptide (VIP) [105].

While low-grade inflammation could also be one of the factors that initiate IBS symptoms in the subset PI-IBS, does low-grade inflammation also occur in sporadic (unselected) IBS? Histopathological examinations of mucosal biopsies from the ileum, caecum, colon and rectum, mostly from IBS-D but even from IBS-C, revealed the infiltration of mast cells and CD3 lymphocytes. Theses findings indicate a possible role of low-grade inflammation in sporadic (unselected) IBS [106-109].

4.6. Abnormalities in the Neuroendocrine System (NES) of the Gut in IBS

4.6.1. The NES of the Gut

A century ago Pavlov proposed that the central nervous system alone controlled the gastrointestinal tract. Since then another local control mechanism has been discovered that is able to control the gut without any central nervous system involvement. This system, called the neuroendocrine system of the gut (NES), consists of two parts: endocrine cells scattered among the epithelial cells of the mucosa facing the gut lumen, and peptidergic, serotonergic and nitric oxide-containing nerves of the enteric nervous system (ENS) in the gut wall (Figure 13) [110]. This system regulates several functions of the gastrointestinal tract, such as motility, secretion, absorption, microcirculation in the gut, local immune defence and cell proliferation [110-116]. This regulatory system includes a large number of neuroendocrine peptides/amines. These bioactive substances exert their effects via an endocrine mode of action (by circulating in the blood to reach distant targets), an autocrine/paracrine mode (local action), via synaptic signalling or via neuroendocrine means (through release from synapses into the circulating blood). The different parts of this system interact and integrate with each other and with afferent and efferent nerve fibres of the central nervous system, in particular the autonomic nervous system.

A large number of endocrine/paracrine cells are dispersed among the epithelial cells of the gut mucosa. These cells constitute the largest endocrine organ in the body and have specialized microvilli that project into the lumen and function as sensors for gut contents and respond to luminal stimuli by releasing hormones that, in general, target other parts of the digestive system (Figure 14) [117-119]. Some of these cells (including somatostatin and PYY cells) have long slender cytoplasmic processes that project to neighbouring cells, making their paracrine action even more efficient. There are at least 14 different populations of endocrine/paracrine cells in the gastrointestinal tract [120]. Different endocrine/paracrine cell types are located in specific areas of the gut, while others [primarily somatostatin and serotonin cells] are found throughout the gut. All of the cell types in the crypt/villus originate from pluripotent stem cells of endodermal origin. This means that enterocytes, Goblet cells, Paneth cells and endocrine/paracrine cells in one crypt/villus are of monoclonal origin [121].

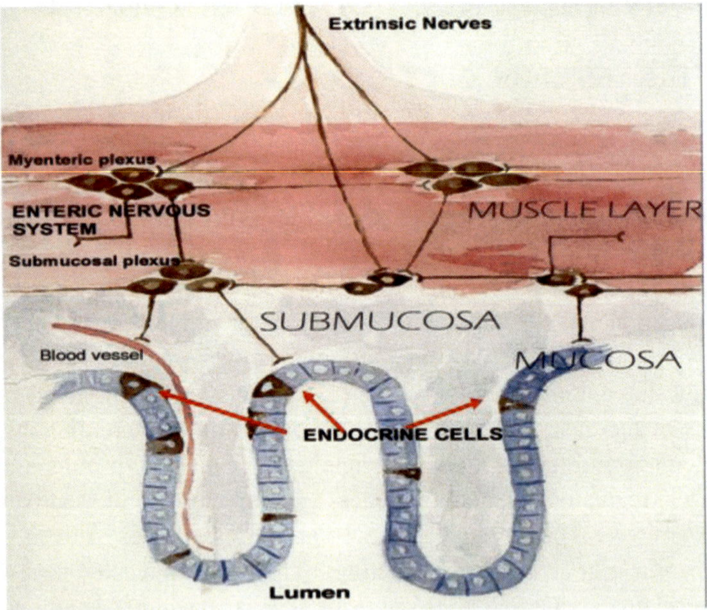

Reproduced from 195.

Figure 13. Schematic drawing to illustrate the neuroendocrine system of the gut.

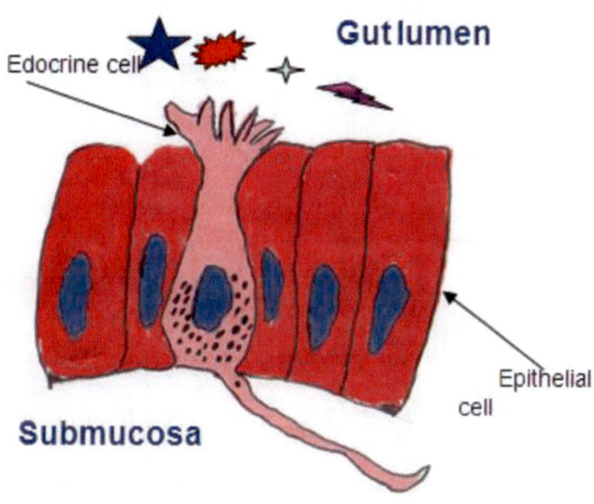

Modified from 195.

Figure 14. Schematic illustration of the endocrine/paracrine cells in the gut. The symbols in the gut lumen from left to right represent carbohydrates, fat, proteins and pressure.

The ENS is by far the most vast and complex component of our peripheral nervous system [122]. A distinguishing feature of the NES is the quantity of neurones, with about 100,000,000 neurones in the human small intestine, which is approximately equal to the number of neurones in the entire spinal cord [123]. Furthermore, the ENS comprises a large variety of neurotransmitters and associated receptors. Almost every known neurotransmitter can be found in the ENS, and most of the receptors associated with these neurotransmitters are also expressed here [123]. More than 20 neuropeptides have been identified in the gut, in addition to the classic transmitters such as acetylcholine, noradrenaline and serotonin [Table 4]. Neurotransmitter action has only been established for a few of these neuropeptides. Many neuropeptides and neurotransmitters are co-localised in the same neurones and one bioactive substance may have different effects on different parts of the gut [116,123]. The gastrointestinal system is the only part of the body with neural reflexes that are entirely housed within the organ. Unlike reflexes associated with the neural control of other organ systems or smooth muscles, complete neural circuits that include sensory neurones, interneurones and motor neurones are contained within the wall of the gut.

Table 4. Overview of the main neuroendocrine peptides/amines in the gastrointestinal tract

Peptide/amine	Amino acid residues	Mode of action	Cellular origin	Action	Released by
Serotonin (5 hydroxyt-Ryptamine)	Amine	Paracrine mediator, transmitter	Enterochromaffin (EC) cells, myenteric and submucosal neurones	Simulates gastric antrum and small intestine as well as gastric emptying and colonic motility; accelerates small intestinal and large intestinal transit.	Noradrenalin; acetylcholine; acidification and intraluminal pressure.
Pancreatic polypeptide (PP)	36	Endocrine	Intestinal PP cell	Inhibits pancreatic secretion; stimulates gastric acid secretion; relaxes the gallbladder and stimulates motility of the stomach and small intestine.	Protein-rich meals.
Neuropeptide Y (NPY)	36	Transmitter, mediator	Myenteric and submucosal neurones	Inhibits pancreatic and intestinal secretion; decreases gastrointestinal motility and is a vasoconstrictor.	Protein-rich meals.
Peptide YY (PYY)	36, 34	Endocrine, paracrine	Intestinal H/L cell	Delays gastric emptying; inhibits gastric and pancreatic secretion and is major ileal brake mediator.	Protein-rich meals.

Peptide/amine	Amino acid residues	Mode of action	Cellular origin	Action	Released by
Gastrin	17, 34	Endocrine	Gastric G-cell	Stimulates gastric acid secretion and histamine release; trophic action on gastric mucosa and stimulates contraction of lower oesophagus (LES) and antrum.	Intraluminal peptides; amino acids; calcium; amines; low pH and prostaglandins. Somatostatin inhibits release.
Cholecystokinin (CCK)	8, 33, 39, 58	Endocrine transmitter?	Intestinal I-cell, myenteric and submucosal neurones	Inhibits gastric emptying; stimulates gallbladder contraction and intestinal motility; stimulates pancreatic exocrine secretion and growth and regulates food intake.	Intraluminal protein and fat and inhibited by somatostatin.
Secretin	27	Endocrine	Intestinal S cell	Stimulates pancreatic bicarbonate and fluid secretion; inhibits gastric emptying and inhibits contractile activity of small and large intestine.	Acidification and inhibited by somatostatin.
Gastric inhibitory peptide (GIP)	42	Endocrine	Small intestinal cells	Incretin; inhibits gastric acid secretion.	Intraluminal glucose; amino acids and fat.

Table 4. (Continued)

Peptide/amine	Amino acid residues	Mode of action	Cellular origin	Action	Released by
Vasoactive polypeptide (VIP)	28	Transmitter, mediator	Myenteric and submucosal neurones	Stimulates gastrointestinal and pancreatic secretion; relaxes smooth muscles in the gut and causes vasodilation.	Serotonin.
Motilin	22	Endocrine	Intestinal M cell	Induces phase III MMC [migrating motor complex]; stimulates gastric emptying and stimulates contraction of LES.	Protein and fat ingestion.
Somatostatin	14, 28	Paracrine, endocrine	Gastric and intestinal D cell, myenteric and submucosal neurones	Inhibits intestinal contraction; and inhibits gut exocrine and neuroendocrine secretion.	Mixed meal and acidification of the stomach.
Peptide/amine	Amino acid residues	Mode of action	Cellular origin	Action	Released by
Ghrelin	28	Endocrine	Gastric oxyntic X/A cell	Ghrelin increases appetite and feeding; stimulates gastric and intestinal motility.	Protein and fat ingestion and suppressed by carbohydrate ingestion.

Peptide/amine	Amino acid residues	Mode of action	Cellular origin	Action	Released by
Enteroglucagon	69	Endocrine	Intestinal L cell	Inhibits gastric and pancreatic secretion.	Intraluminal carbohydrates and fat.
Substance P	11	Transmitter, mediator	Myenteric and submucosal neurones	Stimulates smooth muscle contraction; vasodilator and inhibits gastric acid secretion.	Gut distention
Galanin	30	Transmitter, mediator	Myenteric and submucosal neurones	Inhibits gastric, pancreatic and intestinal secretion delays gastric emptying and intestinal transit and suppresses postprandial release of some neuroendocrine peptides.	Fat
Neurotensin	13	Endocrine transmitter, mediator	Intestinal N cell, myenteric and submucosal neurones	Stimulates pancreatic section; inhibits gastric secretion; delays gastric emptying and stimulates colon motility.	Fat
Nitric oxide (NO)	gas	Transmitter	Myenteric and submucosal neurones	Relaxation of smooth muscle	Activation of protein kinase C alpha and/or epsilon

These circuits are responsible for motility, secretion and vascular tone in the gastrointestinal tract [123].There are two main nerve plexuses in the gut: the myenteric plexus (Auerbach's plexus) located between the longitudinal and the circular muscle layers in the entire gastrointestinal tract, and the submucosal plexus (Meissner's plexus) between the submucosa and the circular muscle Neurones from myenteric ganglia predominantly project to the muscle layer, but also to the mucosa, the submucosal plexus and to other myenteric ganglia. The myenteric plexus contains most of the neurones involved in motility and gastric acid control. Neurones from the submucosal ganglia predominantly project to the mucosa, but also to myenteric ganglia, the circular muscle layer and other submucosal ganglia. These neurones are involved in the control of mucosal fluid transport and vasodilator reflexes. The ganglia of the two plexuses are connected to a continuous meshwork, with the meshwork of the myenteric plexus being more regular. The enteric nervous system receives some input from the central nervous system, but most of the input comes from other enteric neurones [124,125].

4.4.2. Abnormalities in the NES of the Gut in IBS Patients

Available data on the neuroendocrine system of the gut in patients with IBS mainly describe endocrine/paracrine cells in the mucosa as the mucosa is easily biopsied during the standard endoscopic procedure that is performed in these patients. Investigations into the enteric nervous system are considerably more difficult as these require whole wall biopsies to be taken under laparoscopy and this procedure is associated with an increased risk for patients. Moreover, besides the ethical issues this raises, few patients are willing to volunteer to undergo laparoscopy.

Ghrelin is a 28-amino acid peptide hormone that was isolated from the stomach [126] and which may play a role in the pathogenesis of IBS. Ghrelin mostly originates from endocrine cells in the oxyntic mucosa of the stomach, but small amounts are expressed in the small intestine, large intestine and in the arcuated nucleus of the hypothalamus [126,127]. Ghrelin has several functions, including a role in regulating growth hormone [GH] release from the pituitary, where it acts synergistically with the GH-releasing hormone [126,127]. Ghrelin also increases appetite and feeding and plays a major role in energy metabolism [128,129]. Furthermore, ghrelin has been found to accelerate gastric and small and large intestinal motility [130-141]. Ghrelin also has anti-inflammatory actions and protects the gut against a wide range of insults. In the stomach of patients with IBS, the density of ghrelin-immunoreactive cells in the oxyntic mucosa was found to be significantly lower in IBS-constipation patients and significantly higher in IBS-diarrhoea patients compared to healthy controls (Figures 15 and16) [142]. Unexpectedly, the levels of total or active ghrelin in plasma and stomach tissue extracts from IBS patients did not differ from those of healthy subjects [142,143]. Although the density of ghrelin cells is increased in IBS-diarrhoea patients, the synthesis and release of ghrelin may be downregulated in these patients in order to compensate for this. Conversely, ghrelin cell density is decreased in IBS-constipation patients, and therefore ghrelin synthesis and release must be upregulated. One can hypothesise that this compensatory mechanism may be influenced by fatigue, with the subsequent intermittent diarrhoea or constipation seen in IBS patients [142].

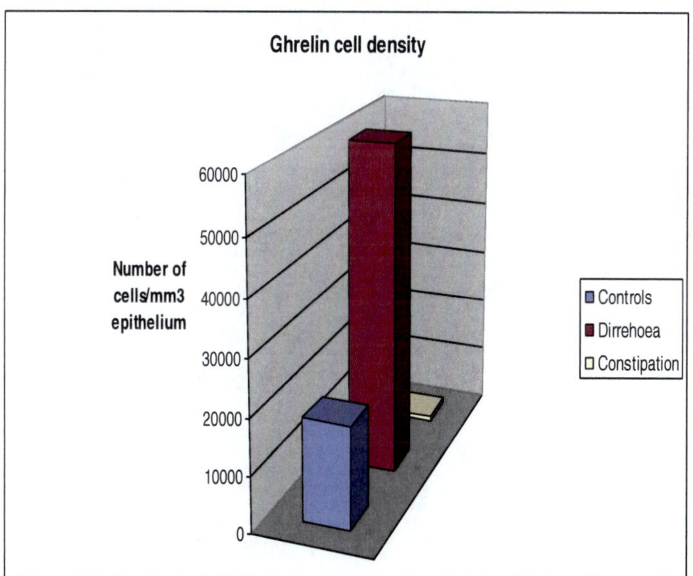

Reproduced from 195.

Figure 15. Ghrelin cell density in the oxyntic mucosa of controls and IBS-diarrhoea and IBS-constipation patients.

The density of neuropeptide-expressing cells is altered in the small intestine of IBS patients. Thus, the density of cells expressing gastric inhibitory polypeptide (GIP) and somatostatin is decreased in patients with both diarrhoea- and constipation-predominant IBS subtypes (Figures 17 and 18).

[144]. The densities of secretin and cholecystokinin (CCK)-expressing cells are decreased in the diarrhoea-predominant subtype, but not in the constipation-predominant subtype. Serotonin cell density has been found to be unchanged in the duodenum of IBS patients, regardless of the subtype. Serotonin cells were previously reported to be affected in the small intestine of IBS patients [145-146]. These peptides all play an important role in secretion and gastric motility.

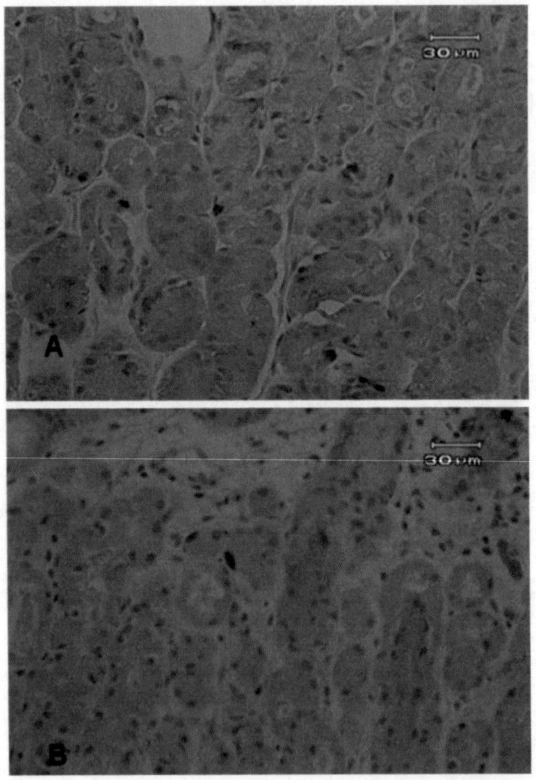

Reproduced from 195.

Figure 16. Ghrelin in the oxyntic mucosa of a healthy subject (A) and in an IBS-C patient (B).

As secretin, GIP and somatostatin inhibit gastric acid secretion [116,117], the reduced density of these cells in the small intestine of IBS patients may result in elevated gastric acid secretion. This could contribute to the high incidence of dyspepsia in IBS patients. Secretin also stimulates pancreatic bicarbonate and fluid secretions [116,117]. The secretion of pancreatic bicarbonate increases the pH of gut contents, which are highly acidic after leaving the stomach, and this is essential for lipid digestion as pancreatic lipase is irreversibly inactivated below pH 4.0 [147]. Cholecystokinin is released in response to nutrients and fatty acids in particular [147,149-147]; it relaxes the proximal stomach in order to increase its reservoir capacity, inhibits gastric emptying and stimulates gall bladder contractions and pancreatic exocrine secretions of digestive enzymes from pancreatic exocrine glands [147]. As secretin and CCK cell densities are low in IBS-diarrhoea patients, this could cause a rapid gastric emptying. It is conceivable that these patients could exhibit a functional pancreatic insufficiency and inadequate emptying of the gall bladder. Indeed, pancreatic enzyme substitution and a low fat-diet have been used in clinical practice for these patients with some success. Furthermore, as secretin inhibits gastric emptying and intestinal motility [116,117], low levels of secretin and CCK could contribute to accelerated gastrointestinal motility and ultimately diarrhoea in these patients [148,149]. It is noteworthy that in IBS, which occurs after acute Giardia infection, the number of CCK and serotonin cells has been reported to be increased [150].

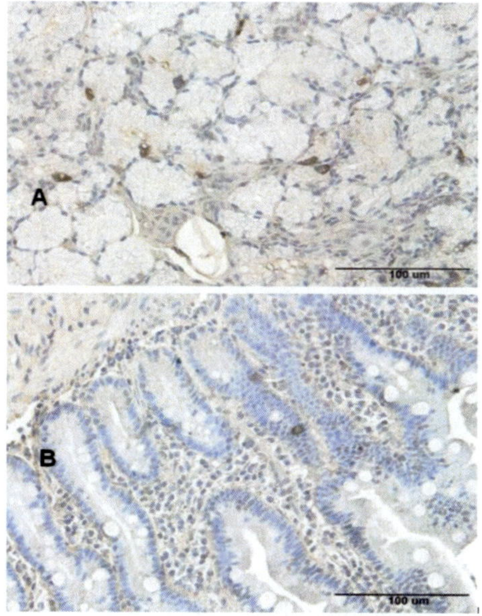

Reproduced from 195.

Figure 17. Cholecystokinin immunoreactive cells in the duodenum of a healthy subject [A] and a patient with IBS-diarrhoea [B].

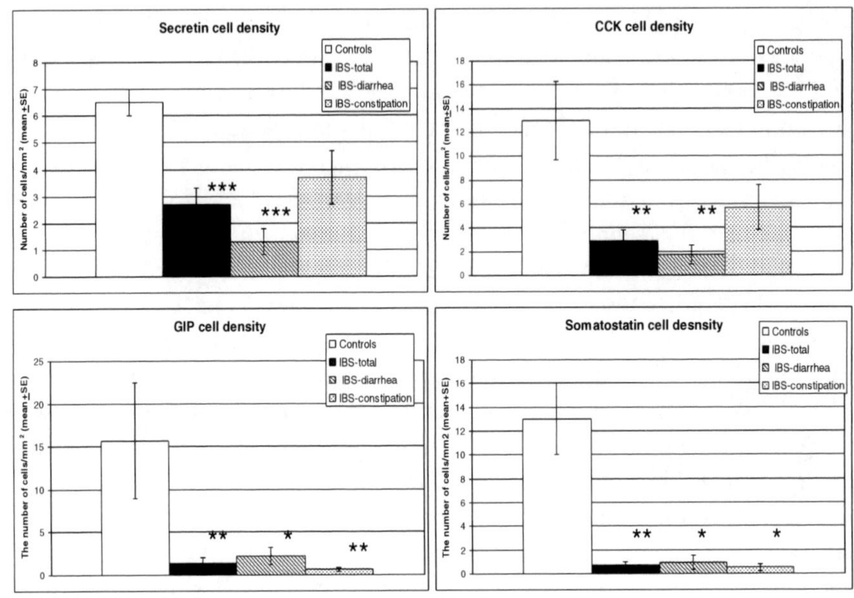

Reproduced from 195.

Figure 18. Secretin, CCK, GIP and somatostatin cell densities in the duodenum of controls and IBS patients. *=P<0.05; **=P<0.01; ***=P>0.001.

In the large intestine, serotonin and polypeptide YY (PYY) cell densities have been found to be low in both IBS-constipation and IBS-diarrhoea patients (Figures 19, 20 and 21) [151]. Furthermore, the mucosal 5-HT concentration has also been reported to be low in IBS patients [149], which is in line with the present observation. About 95% of serotonin in the body is expressed in the gastrointestinal tract and is synthesised by enterochromaffin (EC) cells and sertonergic neurones of the myenteric plexus [150]. Serotonin acts on 5-HT1p receptors, which are located on a subset of inhibitory motor neurones of the myenteric plexus [152,153], and relaxes the stomach via a nitrergic pathway and delays gastric emptying [154-155]. Serotonin secreted by EC cells primarily targets the mucosal projections of primary afferent neurones. These include extrinsic nerves [156-153], which transmit the sensation of nausea and discomfort to the central nervous system, and the mucosal projections of intrinsic primary afferent neurones, which initiate peristaltic and secretory reflexes [160-165]. The secretion of serotonin by myenteric neurones mediates fast and slow excitatory neurotransmission and is involved in regulating gastrointestinal motility [165]. Serotonin stimulates the secretion of chloride and water from the small intestine by acting through 5-HT3 and 5-HT4 receptors [166-171]. Polypeptide YY stimulates the absorption of water and electrolytes and is a major regulator of the "ileal brake" [172-174]. The low density of serotonin cells is likely to reduce motility in the colon of patients with IBS. Low levels of PYY would consequently cause rapid passage from the ileum to the colon and result in watery faeces. As hypothesised, compensation for these low cell numbers could occur through an increase in cellular synthesis and the release of these hormones could result in normal bowel movements in these patients. When this compensator mechanism is affected by fatigue, however, constipation can occur if serotonin secretion is affected, or diarrhoea can occur if PYY secretion is affected [151]. It is noteworthy that in patients with post-infectious IBS of the diarrhoea-predominant type, the number of serotonin cells was found to be increased in the rectum [175-179]. An association between a functional polymorphism in the serotonin transporter [SERT] gene and diarrhoea-predominant IBS was reported [180,181]. Furthermore, it was also reported that tryptophan hydroxylase1 messenger RNA, serotonin transport messenger RNA and serotonin transport immunoreactivity are all reduced in IBS patients [152].

4.5. Hypothesis

This presentation shows that abnormalities in the neuroendocrine peptides/amines of the gut have been reported. These abnormalities would cause disturbances in digestion, gastrointestinal motility and visceral hypersensitivity, and all of these disturbances have been reported in patients with IBS [182-195]. These abnormalities appear to contribute to symptom development and could play a central role in the pathogenesis of IBS.

This presentation also shows that genetic differences have been found between IBS patients and healthy subjects in genes controlling the serotonin signalling system and CCK. Moreover, differences in the diet, intestinal flora and inflammation affect the NES of the gut. The release of different gut hormones depends on the composition and quantity of ingested food. The food content of FODMAPs and fibre, intestinal flora and the subsequent fermentation increase the intestinal osmotic pressure. This change in intestinal pressure would stimulate hormonal release, for example the release of serotonin. Likewise, inflammation and the release of secretory products from immune cells effects hormonal release and the proliferation of gut endocrine cells [196].

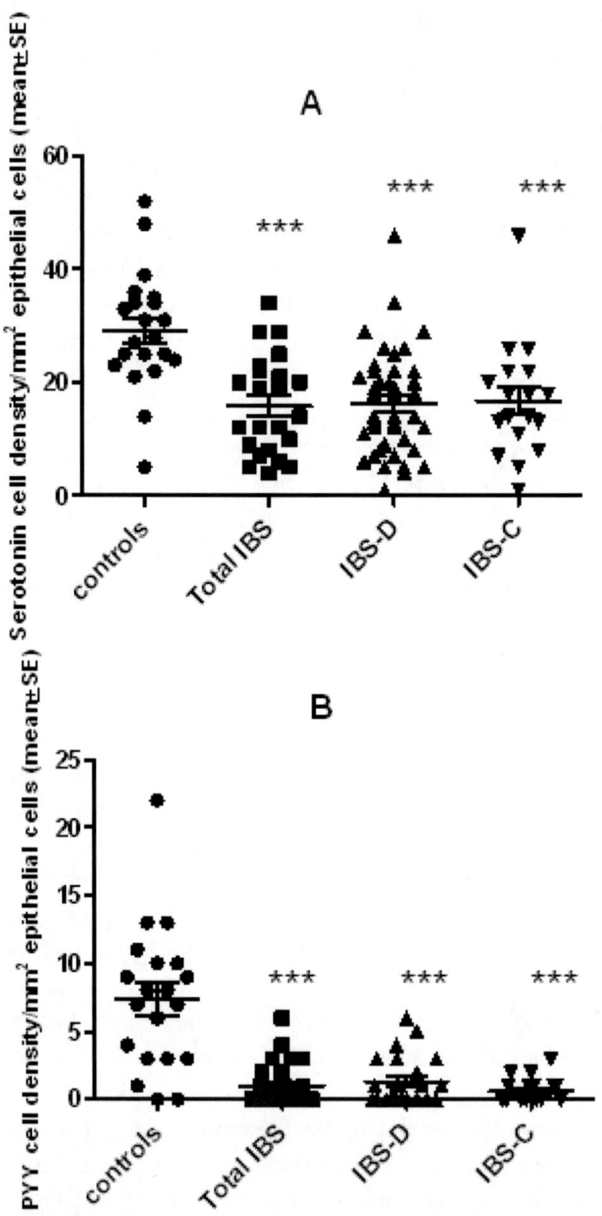

***=P>0.001. Reproduced from 195.

Figure 19. Serotonin [A] and PYY [B] cell densities in the colon of healthy subjects and IBS patients.

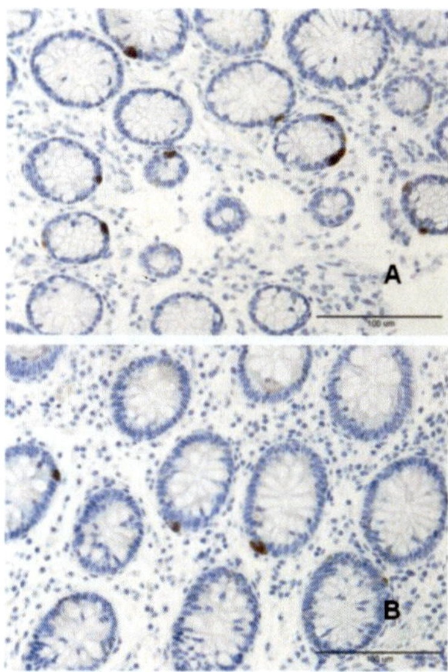

Reproduced from 195.

Figure 20. Serotonin cells in the colon of a healthy control [A] and in a patient with IBS [B].

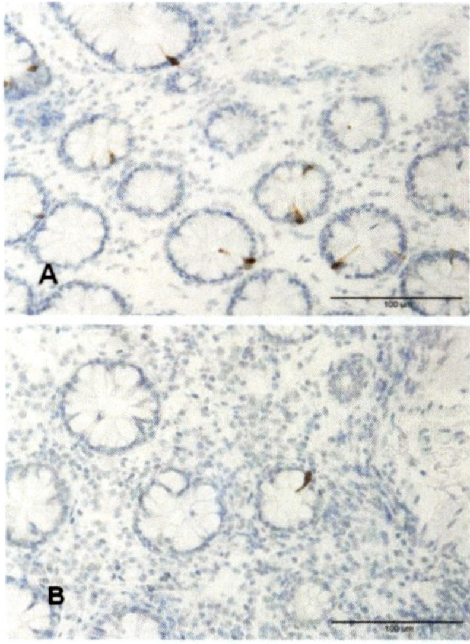

Reproduced from 195.

Figure 21. PYY immunoreactive cells in the colon of a healthy subject [A] and an IBS patient [B].

Therefore, it is feasible to hypothesis (Figure 22) that the cause of IBS is an altered NES. An altered NES would cause abnormal gastrointestinal motility, secretion and sensation. All of these abnormalities are characteristic of IBS. The alteration in NES could be a result of one or more of the following: genetic factors, dietary intake, intestinal flora or low-grade inflammation.

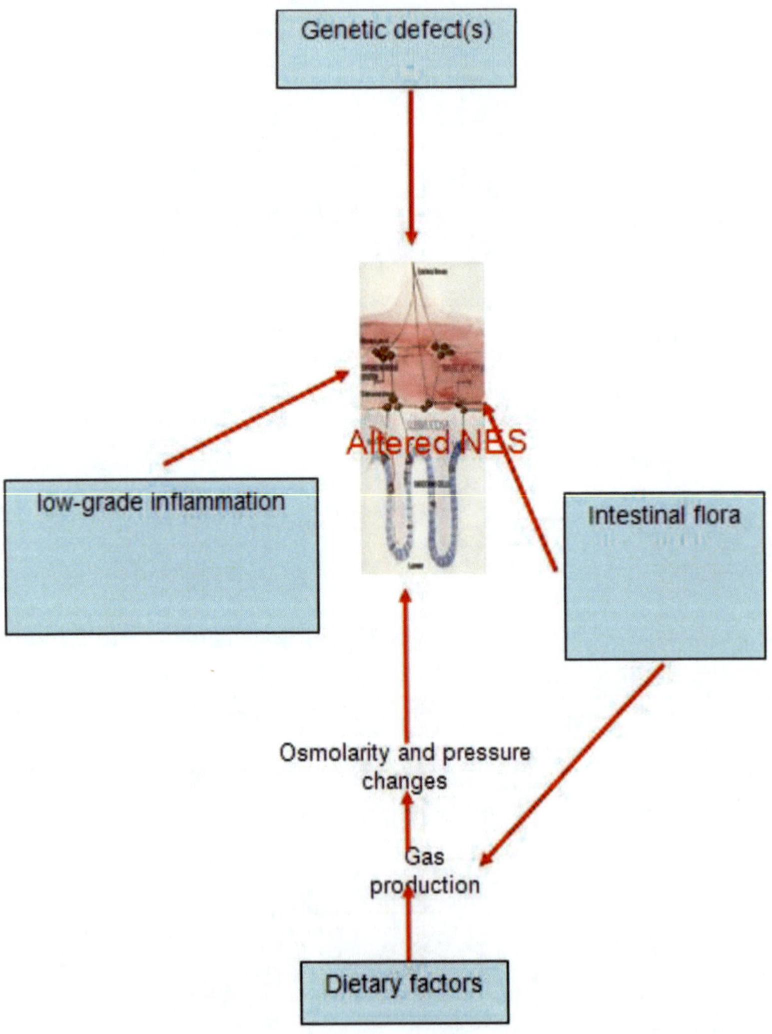

Figure 22. A schematic illustration of the possible pathogenesis of IBS.

References

[1] Locke III GR, Yawn PC, Wollan LJ, Melton III LJ, Lydick E, Talley NJ. Incidence of clinical diagnosis of the irritable bowel syndrome in a United States population. *Aliment Pharmacol Ther* 2004; 19: 1025-1031.

[2] Kessler RC, Berglund P, Demler O, Jin R, Koretz D, Merikangas KR, Rush AJ, Walters EE, Wang PS; National_Comorbidity_Survey Replication. The epidemiology of major depressive disorder: results from the National Comorbidity Survey Replication [NCS-R]. *JAMA* 2003; 289: 3095-3105.

[3] Vandvik PO, Wilhelmsen C, Ihlebaek C, Farup G. Comorbidity of irritable bowel syndrome in general practice: a striking feature with clinical implications. *Aliment Pharmacol Ther* 2004; 20: 1195-1203.

[4] Ihlebaek C, Eriksen HR, Ursin H. Prevalence of subjective health complaints [SHC] in Norway. *Scand J Public Health.* 2002; 30[1]: 20-29.

[5] Kringlen E, Torgersen S, Cramer V. A Norwegian psychiatric epidemiology study. *Am J Psychiatry* 2001; 158: 1091-1098.

[6] Sykes MA, Blanchard EB, Lackner J, Keefer L, Krasner S. Psychopathology in irritable bowel syndrome: support for a psychophysiological model. *J Behav Med* 2003; 26: 361-372.

[7] Pan G, Lu S, Ke M, Han S, Guo H, Fang X. Epidemiologic study of the irritable bowel syndrome in Beijing: stratified randomized study by cluster sampling. *Chin Med J [Engl]* 2000; 113: 35-39.

[8] Bennett EJ, Piesse C, Palmer K, Badcock CA, Tennant CC, Kellow JE. Functional gastrointestinal disorders: psychological, social, and somatic features. *Gut* 1998; 42: 414-420.

[9] Drossman DA, Camilleri M, Mayer EA, Whitehead WE. AGA technical review on irritable bowel syndrome. *Gastroenterology* 2002; 123: 2108-2131.

[10] North CS, Downs D, Clouse RE, Alrakawi A, Dokucu ME, Cox J, Spitznagel EL, Alpers DH. The presentation of irritable bowel syndrome in the context of somatization disorder. *Clin Gastroenterol Hepatol* 2004; 2: 787-795.

[11] Whitehead WE, Palsson O, Jones KR. Systematic review of the comorbidity of irritable bowel syndrome with other disorders: what are the causes and implications? *Gastroenterology* 2002; 122: 1140-1156.

[12] Spiller R, Aziz Q, Creed F, Emmanuel A, Houghton L, Hungin P, Jones R, Kumor D, Rubin G, Trudgill N, Whorwell P. Guidelines on the

irritable bowel syndrome: mechanisms and practical management. *Gut* 2007; 56: 1770-1798.

[13] Gershon MD, Tack J. The serotonin signaling system: from basic understanding to drug development for functional GI disorders. *Gastroenterology* 2007; 132: 397-414.

[14] Drossman DA, Leserman J, Nachman G,Li Z, Gluck H,Toomey TC. Sexual and physical abuse in women with functional or organic gastrointestinal disorders. *Ann Intern Med* 1990; 113: 828-833.

[15] Talley NJ, Helgeson SI, Zinsmeister AR, Melton LJ III. Gastrointestinal tract symptoms and self reported abuse: a population-based study. *Gastroenterology* 1994; 107: 1040-1049.

[16] Talley NJ, Fett SL, Zinsmeister AR. Self-reported abuse and gastrointestinal diseases in outpatients associated with irritable bowel syndrome-type symptoms. *Am J Gastroenterol* 1995; 90: 366-371.

[17] Walker EA, Gelfand AN, Gelfand MD, Kanton WJ. Pachiatric diagnosis, sexual and victimisation, and disability in patients with irritable bowel syndrome or inflammatory bowel disease. *Pyschol Med* 1995; 25: 1259-1267.

[18] Drossman DA. Abuse, trauma, and GI illness: is there a link? *Am J Gastroenterol* 2011; 106: 14-25.

[19] Drossman DA, Li Z, Toner BB, Diamant NE, Creed FH, Thompson D, Read NW, Babbs C, Barreiro M, Bank L, et al. Functional bowel disorders. A multicenter comparison of health status and development of illness severity index. *Dig Dis Sci* 1995; 40: 986-995.

[20] Leserman J, Li Z, Drossman DA, Toomey TC, Nachman G, Glogau L. Impact of sexual and physical abuse dimensions on health status: development of an abuse severity measure. *Psychosom Med* 1997; 59: 152-160.

[21] Talley NJ, Boyes PM, Jones M. Is the association between irritable bowel syndrome and abuse explained by neuroticism? A population based study. *Gut* 1998; 42: 47-53.

[22] Whitehead WE, Crowell MD, Davidoff AL, Palsson OS, Schuster MM. Pain from rectal distension in women with irritable bowel syndrome: relationship to sexual abuse. *Dig Dis Sci* 1997; 42: 796-804.

[23] Ringel Y, Whitehead WE, Toner BB, Diamant NE, Hu Y, Jia H, Bangdiwala SI, Drossman DA. Sexual and physical abuse are not associated with rectal hypersensitivity in patients with irritable bowel syndrome. *Gut* 2004; 53: 838-842.

[24] Creed F, Guthrie E. Psychological factors in the irritable bowel syndrome. *Gut* 1987; 28: 1307-1318.

[25] Hotoleanu C, Popp R, Trifa AP, Nedelcu L, Dumitrascu DL. Genetic determination of irritable bowel syndrome. *World J Gastroenterol* 2008; 14: 6636-6640.

[26] Whorwell PJ, McCallum M, Creed FH, Roberts CT. Non-colonic features of irritable bowel syndrome. *Gut* 1986; 27: 37-40.

[27] Locke GR 3rd, Zinsmeister AR, Talley NJ, Fett SL, Melton LJ 3rd. Familial association in adults with functional gastrointestinal disorders. *Mayo Clin Proc* 2000; 75: 907-912.

[28] Kalantar JS, Locke GR 3rd, Zinsmeister AR, Beighley CM, Talley NJ. Familial aggregation of irritable bowel syndrome: a prospective study. *Gut* 2003; 52: 1703-1707.

[29] Kanazawa M, Endo Y, Whitehead WE, Kano M, Hongo M, Fukudo S. Patients and nonconsulters with irritable bowel syndrome reporting a parental history of bowel problems have more impaired psychological distress. *Dig Dis Sci* 2004; 49: 1046-1053.

[30] Morris-Yates A, Talley NJ, Boyce PM, Nandurkar S, Andrews G. Evidence of a genetic contribution to functional bowel disorder. *Am J Gastroenterol* 1998; 93: 1311-1317.

[31] Levy RL, Jones KR, Whitehead WE, Feld SI, Talley NJ, Corey LA. Irritable bowel syndrome in twins: heredity and social learning both contribute to etiology. *Gastroenterology* 2001; 121: 799-804.

[32] Lembo A, Zaman M, Jones M, Talley NJ. Influence of genetics on irritable bowel syndrome, gastro-oesophageal reflux and dyspepsia: a twin study. *Aliment Pharmacol Ther* 2007; 25: 1343-1350.

[33] Wojczynski MK, North KE, Perdersen NL, Sullivan. Irritable bowel syndrome: a co-twin control analysis. *Am J Gastroenterol* 2007; 102: 2220-2229.

[34] Bengtson MB, Ronning T, Vatn MH, Harris JR. Irritable bowel syndrome in twins: genes and environment. *Gut* 2006; 55: 1754-1759.

[35] Mohammed I, Cherkas LF, Riley SA, Spector TD, Trudgill NJ. Genetic influences in irritable bowel syndrome: a twin study. *Am J Gastroenterol* 2005; 100: 1340-1344.

[36] Yeo A, Boyd P, Lumsden S, Saunders T, Handley A, Stubbins M, Knaggs A, Asquith S, Taylor I, Bahari B, Crocker N, Rallan R, Varsani S, Montgomery D, Alpers DH, Dukes GE, Purvis I, Hicks GA. Association between a functional polymorphism in the serotonin

[61] Zar S, Benson MJ, Kumar D. Food specific serum IgG4 and IgE titers to common food antigens in irritable syndrome. *Am J Gastroenterol* 2005; 100: 1550-1557.

[62] Park MI, Camilleri M. Is there a role of food allergy in irritable bowel syndrome and functional dyspepsia? A systematic review. *Neurogastroenterol Motil* 2006; 18: 595-607.

[63] Uz E, Türkay C, Aytac S, Bavbek N. Risk factors for irritable bowel syndrome in turkish population: role of food allergy. *J Clin Gastroenterol* 2007; 41: 380-383.

[64] Dainese R, Galliani EA, De Lazzari F, Di Leo V, Naccarato R. Discrepancies between reported food intolerance and sensitization test findings in irritable bowel syndrome patients. Amr J Gastroenterol 1999; 94: 1892-1897.

[65] Bischoff S, Crowe SE. Gastrointestinal food allergy: New insights into pathophysiology and clinical perspectives. Gastroenterology 2005; 128: 1089-1113.

[66] Murch S. Allergy and intestinal dysmotility-Evidence of genuine causal linkage? Curr Opin Gastroenterol 2006; 22: 664-668.

[67] Gui XY. Mast cells. A possible link between psychological stress, enteric infection, food allergy and gut hypersensitivity in the irritable bowel syndrome. J Gastroenterol Hepatol 1998; 13: 980-989.

[68] Spiller R, Campbell E. Post-infectious irritable bowel syndrome. Curr Opin Gastroenterol 2006; 22: 13-17.

[69] Walker MM, Talley NJ. Functional disorders and the potential role of esinophils. Gastroenterol Clin North Am 2008; 37: 383-395.

[70] Peptipierre M, Gumowski P, Girard JP. Irritable bowel syndrome and hypersensitivity to food. Ann Allergy 1985; 54: 538-540.

[71] Tobin MC, Moparty B, Farhadi A, DeMeo MT, Bansal PJ, Kashavarzian A. Atopic irritable bowel syndrome: A novel subgroup of irritable bowel syndrome with allergic manifestations. *Ann Allergy Asthma Immunol* 2008; 100: 49-53.

[72] Zar S, Mincher L, Benson MJ, Kumar D. Food specific IgG4 antibody-guided exclusion diet improves symptoms and rectal compliance in irritable bowel syndrome. *Scand J Gastroenterol* 2005; 40: 800-807.

[73] Akinson W, Sheldon TA, Sheath N, Whorwell PJ. Food elimination based on IgG antibodies in irritable bowel syndrome: a randomised controlled trial. *Gut* 2004; 53: 1459-1464.

[74] Zar S, Kumar D, Benson MJ. Food hypersensitivity and irritable bowel syndrome. *Aliment Pharmacol Ther* 2001; 15: 439-449.

[75] Whorwell PJ. The growing case for an immunological component to irritable bowel syndrom. Clin Exp Allergy 2007; 37: 805-807.

[76] Hunter JO. Food elimination in IBS: the case for IgG testing remains doubtful. Gut 2005; 54: 1203.

[77] Taufel M, Biedermann T, Rapps N, Hausteiner C,Henningsen P, Enck P, Zipfel S. Psychological burden of food allergy. World J Gastroenterol 2007; 13: 3456-3465.

[78] Beyer K, Teuber SS. Food allergy diagnostic: Scientific and unproven procedures. *Curr Opin Allergy Clin Immunol* 2005; 5: 261-266.

[79] Choung RS. Food allergy and intolerances in IBS. *Gastroenterol Hepatol* 2006; 2: 756-760.

[80] Ortolani C, Bruijinzeel-Koomen C, Bengtsson U, Bindslev-Jensen C, Björkstén B, Høst A, Ispano M, Jarish R, Madsen C, Nekam K, Paganelli R, Poulsen LK, Wüthrich B . Controversial aspects of adverse reactions of food. European Academy of Allergology and Clinical Immunology [EAACI] reactions to food subcommittee. *Allergy* 1999; 54: 27-45.

[81] Fissora CI. Koch KL. Symptom overlap and comorbidity of irritable bowel syndrome with other conditions. *Curr Gastroenterol Rep* 2005; 7: 264-271.

[82] Young E, Stoneham MD, Petruckevitch A, Barton J, Rona R. A population study of food intolerance. *Lancet* 1994; 343:1127-1130.

[83] Locke GR, Zinsmeister AR, Talley NJ, Fett SL, Melton LJ. Risk factors for irritable bowel syndrome: role of analgesics and food sensitivities. *Am J Gastroenterol* 2000; 95: 157-165.

[84] Bischoff SC, Hermann MP. Prevalence of adverse reactions to food in patients with gastrointestinal disease. Allergy 1996, 51: 811-818.

[85] Nanda R, James R, Smith H, Dudley CR, Jewell DP. Food intolerance and irritable bowel syndrome. *Gut* 1989; 30: 1099-1104.

[86] Jones VA, Shorthouse M, Hunter JO. Food intolerance: a major factor in the pathogenesis of irritable bowel syndrome. *Lancet* 1982; 2: 1115-1117.

[87] Bhat K, Harper A, Gorard DA. Perceived food and drug allergies in functional and organic gastrointestinal disorders. *Aliment Pharmacol Ther* 2002; 16: 969-973.

[88] Bijkerk CJ, deWit NJ, Stalman WA, Knottnerus JA, Hoes AW, Muris JW. Irritable bowel syndrome in primary care: The patients and doctors views on symptoms, etiology and management. *Can J Gastroenterol* 2003; 17: 363-368.

[89] Ford AC, Talley NJ, Spiegel BM, Foxx-Orenstein AE, Schiller L, Quigley EM, Moayyedi P. Effect of fibres, antispasmodics, and peppermint oil in the treatment of irritable bowel syndrome: systematic review and meta-analysis. *BMJ* 2008; 337: a2313.

[90] Francis CY, Whorwell PJ. Bran and irritable bowel syndrome: time for reappraisal. *Lancet* 1994; 344: 39-40.

[91] Bijkerk CJ, deWit NJ, Muris JW, Whorwell PJ, Knottnerus JA, Hoes AW. Soluble or insoluble fibre in irritable bowel syndrome in primary care? Randomised placebo controlled trial. *BMJ* 2009; 339: b3154.

[92] Quigley EM. Probiotics and digestive health. 2008; Health point press.

[93] Kassinen A, Kroguius-Kurikka L, Mäkivuokko H, , Rinttilä T, Paulin L, Corander J, Malinen E, Apajalahti J, Palva A. The fecal microbiota of irritable bowel syndrome patients differs significantly from that of healthy subjects. *Gastroenterology* 2007; 133: 24-33.

[94] Spiller R. Review article: probiotics and prebiotics in irritable bowel syndrome. *Ailment Pharmacol Ther* 2008; 28: 385-396.

[95] Brenner DM, Moeller MJ, Chey WD,Schoenfeld PS. The utility of probiotics in the treatment of irritable bowel syndrome: a systematic review. *Am J Gastroenterol* 2009; 104: 1033-1049.

[96] Levy RL, Linde JA, Feld KA, Crowell MD, Jeffery RW. The association of gastrointestinal symptoms with weight diet and exercise in weight-loss program participants. *Clin Gastroenterol Hepatol* 2005; 2: 992-6.

[97] Spiller RC. Role of infection in irritable bowel syndrome. *J Gastroenterol* 2007; 42 [Suppl XVII]: 41-47.

[98] Spiller R, Garsed K. Infection, inflammation, and irritable bowel syndrome. *Dig Liver Dis* 2009; 41: 844-849.

[99] Spiller R, Garsed K. P ostinfectious irritable bowel syndrome. *Gastroenterology* 2009; 136: 1979-1988.

[100] Neal KR, Hebden J, Spiller R. Prevalence of gastrointestinal symptoms six month after bacterial gastroenteritis and risk factors for development of irritable bowel syndrome: postal survey of patients. *Br Med J* 1997; 314: 779-782.

[101] Spiller RC, Jenkins D, Thornley JP, Hebden JM, Wright T, Skinner M, Neal KR. Increased rectal mucosal enteroenocrine cells, T lymphocytes, and increased gut permeability following acute Campylobacter enteritis and in post-dysenteric irritable bowel syndrome. *Gut* 2000; 47: 804-811.

[102] Spiller R. Serotonin, inflammation, and IBS: fitting the jigsaw together? *Pediatr Gastroenterol Nutr* 2007; 45[Suppl. 2]: S115-119.

[103] Khan WI, Ghia JE. Gut hormones: emerging role in immune activation and inflammation. *Clin Exp Immunol* 2010; 161: 19-27.

[104] Yang GB, Lackner AA. Proximity between 5HT secreting enteroenocrine cells and lymphocytes in gut mucosa of rhesus macaques [Macaca mulatta] is suggesting a role for enterochromaffin cell 5HT in mucosal immunity. *J Neuroimmunol* 2004; 146: 46-49.

[105] Qian B-F. An experimental study on the interaction between the neuro-endocrine and immune systems in the gastrointestinal tract. Umeå University Medical Dissertations 2001; No 719: 1-62.

[106] Wetson AP, Biddle WL, Bhatia PS, Miner PB Jr. Terminal ileal mucosal mast cells in irritable bowel syndrome. Dig Dis Sci 1993; 38: 1590-1595.

[107] O'Sullivan M, Clayton N, Breslin NP, Herman I, Bountra C, McLaren A, O'Morain CA. Increased mast cells in the irritable bowel syndrome. *Neurogastroenterol Motil* 2000; 12: 449-457.

[108] Dunlop SP, Jenkins D, Neal KR, Spiller RC. Clinical and histological features of post-infectious IBS: relative importance of enterochromaffin cell hyperplasia, anxiety and depression. Gastroenterology 2003; 125: 1651-1659.

[109] Barbara G, Stanghellini V, De Giorgio R, Cremon C, Cottrell GS, Santini D, Pasquinelli G, Morselli-Labate AM, Grady EF, Bunnett NW, Collins SM, Corinaldesi R. Activated mast cells in proximity to colonic nerves correlated with abdominal pain in irritable bowel syndrome. *Gastroenterology* 2004; 126: 693-702.

[110] El-Salhy M. The possible role of the gut neuroendocrine system in diabetes gastroenteropathy. *Histol Histopathol* 2002; 17: 1153-1161.

[111] Allescher HD. Postulated physiological and pathophysiological on motility. In Daniel E, Ed. Neuropeptides function in gastrointestinal tract. Boca Raton: CRC Press 1991; pp. 309-400.

[112] Debas HT, Mulvihill SJ. Neuroendocrine design of the gut. *Am J Surg* 1991; 161: 243-249.

[113] Ekblad E, Håkansson R, Sundler F. Microanatomy and chemical coding of peptide -containing neurones in the digestive tract. . In Daniel E, Ed. Neuropeptids function in gastrointestinal tract. Boca Raton: CRC Press 1991; pp 131-180.

[114] Rangachari PK. Effects of neuropeptides on intestinal transport. In Daniel E, Ed. Neuropeptids function in gastrointestinal tract. Boca Raton: CRC Press 1991; pp. 429-446.

[115] Mc Conalogue K, Furness JB. Gastrointestinal transmitters. *Baollieres Clin Endocrinol Meatabol* 1994; 8: 51-76.

[116] Goyal PK, Hirano I. Mechanisms of disease: the enteric nervous system. *N Engl J Med* 1996; 334: 1106-1115.

[117] El-Salhy M. Ghrelin in gastrointestinal diseases and disorders: A possible role in the pathophsiology and clinical implications. *J Mol Med* 2009; 24: 727-732.

[118] El-Salhy M. Gut neuroendocrine system in diabetes gastroenteropathy, In Ashley M, Ed. Possible role in pathophysiology and clinical implications. Focus on Diabetes Research. New York: Nova Science Publisher 2006; pp.79-102.

[119] Sandström O. Age-related changes in the neuroendocrine system of the gut: a possible role in the pathogenesis of gastrointestinal disorders in the elderly. Umeå University Medical Dissertations 1999 No 617:1-46.

[120] Leibowitz SF, Akabyashi A, Wang J, Alexander JT, Dourmashkin JT, Chang GQ. Increased caloric intake on a fat-rich diet: role of ovarian steroids and galanin in the medial preoptic and paraventricular nuclei and anterior pituitary of female rats. *J Neuroendocrinol* 2007; 19: 753-766.

[121] Miller LJ. gastrointestinal hormones and receptors. In Yamada T, Alpers DH, Laine L, Owyang C, Powell DW, Eds. Textbook of gastroenterology, 3rd edn.   Philadephian, PA: Lippincott-Williams and Wilkins, 1999; pp. 35-66.

[122] Buchan AM. Nutrient tasting and signaling mechanisms in the gut III. Endocrine cell recognition of luminal nutrients. *Am Physiol* 1999; 277: G1103-1107.

[123] Rindi G, Kloppel G. Endocrine tumors of the gut and pancreas tumor biology and classification. *Neuroendocrinology* 2004; 80[Suppl. 2]: 12-15.

[124] Sandström O, El-Salhy M. Age-related changes in the neuroendocrine system of the gut. A possible role in the pathogenesis of gastrointestinal disorders in the elderly. *Upsala J Med Sci* 2001; 106: 81-97.

[125] Lundgren O. Enteric nerves and diarrhoea. *Pharmacol Toxicol* 2002; 90: 109-120.

[126] Kojima M, Hosoda H, Date J, Nakazato M, Matsuo H, Kangawa K. Ghrelin is growth-hormone-releasing acetylated peptide from stomach. Nature 1999; 402: 656-660.

[127] Date Y, Kojima M, Hosoda H, Sawaguchi A, Mondal MS, Suganuma T, Matsukura S, Kangawa K, Nakazato M. Ghrelin, a novel growth

hormone-releasing acetylated peptide, is synthesized in a distinct endocrine cell type in the gastrointestinal tracts of rats and humans. *Endocrinology* 2000; 141: 4255-4261.

[128] Hataya Y, Akamizu T, Takaya K, Kanamoto N, Ariyasu H, Saijo M, Moriyama K, Shimatsu A, Kojima M, Kangawa K, Nakao K. A low dose of ghrelin stimulates growth hormone [GH] release synergistically with GH-releasing hormone in humans. *J Clin Endocrinol Metab* 2001; 86: 4552-4558.

[129] Wren AM, Seal LJ, Cohen M, Brynes AE, Frost GS, Murphy KG, Dhillo WS, Ghatei MA, Bloom SR. Ghrelin enhances appetite and increases food intake in humans. *J Clin Endocrinol Metab* 2001; 86: 5992-5998.

[130] Hosoda H, Kojima M and Kangawa K. Ghrelin and the regulation of food intake and energy balance. *Mol Interv* 2002; 8: 494-503.

[131] Masuda Y, Tanaka T, Inomata N, Ohmura N, Tanaka S, Itoh Z. Ghrelin stimulates gastric acid secretion and motility in rats. *Biochem Biophys Res Commun* 2000; 276: 905-908.

[132] Fujino K, Inui A, Asakawa A, Kihara N, Fujimura M, Fujimiya M. Ghrelin induces fasted motor activity of the gastrointestinal tract in conscious fed rats. *J Physiol* 2003; 550: 227-240.

[133] Dornonville de la Cour C, Lindstrom E, Noren P, Hakansson R. Ghrelin stimulates gastric emptying but without effect on acidsecretion and gastric endocrine cells. *Regul Pept* 2004; 120: 23-32.

[134] Fukuda H, Mizuta Y, Isomoto H, Takeshima F, Ohnita K, Ohba K. Ghrelin enhances gastric motility through directstimulation of intrinsic neural pathway and capsaicin-sensitive afferent neurones in rats. *Scand J Gastroenterol* 2004; 39:1209-1214.

[135] Levin F, Edholm T, Schmidt PT, Gryback P, Jacobsson H, Dergerblad M. Ghrelin stimulates gastric emptying and hunger in normal weight humans. *J Clin Endocrinol* Metab 2006; 91: 3279-3280.

[136] Tack J, Deportere I, Bischops R, Delporte C, Coulie B, Meulemans A: Influence of ghrelin on interdigestive gastrointestinal motility in humans. *Gut* 2006; 55: 327-333.

[137] Ariga H, Tsukamoto K, Chen C, Mantyh C, Pappas TN, Takahashi T. Endogenus acyl ghrelin is involved in mediating spontaneous phase III-like contractions in the rat stomach. *Neurogastroenterol Motil* 2007; 19: 675-680.

[138] Ariga H, Nakade Y, Tsukamoto K, Imai K, Chen C, Mantyh C, Pappas TN, Takahashi T. Ghrelin accelerates gastric emptying via an early

manifestation of antro-pyloric coordination in conscious rats. *Regul Pep* 2008; 146: 112-116.

[139] Tumer C, Oflazoglu HD, Obay BD, Kelle M, Tasdemir E. Effects of ghrelin on gastric myoelectrical activity and gastric emptying in rats. Regul Pep 2008; 146: 26-32.

[140] Edholm T, Levin F, Hellerstrom PM, Schmidt PT. Ghrelin stimulates motility in the small intestine of rats. Regul Pep 2004; 121: 25-30.

[141] Tabbe JJ, Mornga S, Tebbe CG, Oertmann E, Arnold R, Chafer K. Ghrelin-induced stimulation of colonic propulsion is dependent on hypothalamic neuropeptides Y1- and corticotrophin-releasing factor 1 receptor activation. *J Neuroendocrinol* 2005; 17: 570-576.

[142] El-Salhy M, Lillebö E, Reinemo A, Salmelid L. Ghrelin in patients with irritable bowel syndrome. *Int J Mol Med* 2009; 23: 703-707.

[143] Sjölund K, Ekman R, Wierup N. Covariation of plasma ghrelin and motilin in   irritable bowel syndrome. *Peptides* 2010; 31: 1109-12.

[144] El-Salhy M, Vaali K, Dizdar V, Hausken T. Abnormal small intestinal endocrine cells in patients with irritable bowel syndrome. *Dig Dig Sci* 2010; 55: 3508-3513.

[145] Wang SH, Dong L, Luo JY, Gong J, Li L, Lu XL, Han SP. Decreased expression of serotonin in the jejenum and increased numbers of mast cells in the terminal ileum in patients with irritable bowel syndrome. *World J Gastroenterol* 2007; 13: 6041-6047.

[146] Park JH, Rhee P-L, Kim G, Lee JH, Kim YH, Kim JJ, Rhee JC, Song SY. Enteroendocrine cell counts correlated with visceral hypersensitivity in patients with diarrhoea-predominant irritable bowel syndrome. *Neurogastroenterol Motil.* 2006; 18: 539-546.

[147] Camilleri M. Integrated upper gastrointestinal response to food intake. *Gastroenterology* 2006; 131: 640-658.

[148] Lal S, McLaughlin J, Barlow J, D'Amato M, Giacovelli G, Varro A, Dockray GJ, Thompson DG. Cholecystokinin pathways modulate sensations induced by gastric distension in humans. *Am J Physiol* 2004; 287: G72-G79.

[149] Moran TH , Ladenheim EE , Schwartz GJ. Within-meal gut feedback signaling . *Int J Obes Relat Metab Disord.* 2001; 25[Suppl 5]: S39-S41.

[150] Dizdar V, Spiller R, Hanevik K, Gilja OH, El-Salhy M, Hausken T. Relative importance of CCK [cholecystokinin] and 5-HT [serotonin] in Giardia-induced Post-infectious IBS. *Aliment Pharmacol Ther* 2010; 31: 883-891.

[151] El-Salhy M, Gundersen D, Østgaard H, Lomholt-Beck B, Hatlebakk JG, Hausken T. Low densities of serotonin and peptide YY cells in the colon of patients with irritable bowel syndrome. 2011; *Dig Dis Sci*, DOI: 10.1007/s10620-011-1948-8.

[152] Coates MD, Mahoney CR, Linden DR, Sampson JE, Chen J, Blaszyk H, Crowell MD, Sharkey KA, Gershon MD, Mawe GM, Moses PL. Molecular defects in mucosal serotonin content and decreased serotonin reuptake transporter in ulcerative colitis and irritable bowel syndrome. *Gastroenterology* 2004; 126: 1657-1664.

[153] Gershon MD, Tack J. The serotonin signaling system: from basic understanding to drug development for functional GI disorders. *Gastroenterology* 2007; 132: 397-414.

[154] Tack JF, Janssens J, Vantrappen G, Wood JD. Actions of 5-hydroxytryptamine on myenteric neurones in gastric antrum of guinea pig. *Am J physiol* 1992; 263: G838-G846.

[155] Michel K, Sann H, Schaff C, Schemann M. Subpopulations of gastric neurones are differentially activated via distinct serotonin receptors: projection, neurochemical coding, and functional implications. *J Neurosci* 1997; 17: 8009-8017.

[156] Tack J, Coulie B,Wilmer A, Andrioli A, Janssens J. Influence of sumartriptan on gastric fundus tone and on the presence of gastric distension in human. *Gut* 2000; 46: 468-473.

[157] Tack J, Demedts I, Dehondt G, Caenepeel P, Fischler B, Zandecki M, Janssens J. Clinical and pathophysiological characteristics of acute-onset of unctional dyspepsia. *Gastroenterology* 2002; 122: 1738-1747.

[158] Coulie B, Tack J, Maes B, Geypens B, De Roo, M, Jensens J. Sumatriptan, a selective 5-HT 1 receptor agonist, induces a lag phase for gastric emptying of liquids in humans. *Am J Physiol* 1997; 272: G902-G908.

[159] Sugiuar T, Bielefeldt K, Gebhart GF. TRPV1 function in mouse colon sensory neurons is enhanced by metabotropic 5-hydroxytryptamine receptor activation. *J Neurosci* 2004; 24: 9521-9530.

[160] Hillsley K, Kirkup AJ, Grundy D. Direct and indirect actions of 5-hydroxytryptamine on the discharge of mesenteric afferent fibers innervating the rat jejunum. *J Physiol* [Lond] 1998; 506: 551-561.

[161] Hillsley K, Grundy D. Sensitivity to 5-hydroxytryptamine in different afferent subpopulations within mesenteric nerves supplying the rat jejunum. *J Physiol* [Lond] 1998; 509: 717-727.

[162] Grundy D, Blackshaw LA, Hillsley K. Role of 5-hydroxytryptamine in gastrointestinal chemosensitivity. *Dig Dis Sci* 1994; 39[Suppl 12]: S44-S47.

[163] Blackshaw LA, Grundy D. Effects of 5-hydroxytryptamine on discharge of vagal mucosal afferent fibres from the upper gastrointestinal tract of the ferret. *J Auton Nerv Syst* 1993; 45: 41-50.

[164] Kirchgessner AL, Tamir H, Gershon MD. Identification and stimulation by serotonin of intrinsic sensory neurons of the submucosal plexus of the guinea pig gut: activity-induced expression of Fos immunoreactivity. *J Neurosci* 1992; 12: 235-249.

[165] Kirchgessner AL, Liu M-T, Gershon MD. In situ identification and visualization of neurons that mediate enteric and enteropancreatic reflexes. *J Comp Neurol* 1996; 371: 270-286.

[166] Pan H, Gershon MD. Activation of intrinsic afferent pathways in submucosal ganglia of the guinea pig small intestine. *J Neurosci* 2000; 20: 3295-3309.

[167] Sidhu M, Cooke HJ. Role for 5-HT and ACh in submucosal reflexes mediating colonic secretion. Am J *Physiol Gastointest Liver Physiol* 1995; 269: G346-G351.

[168] Cooke HJ, Sidhu M, Wang Y-Z. 5-HT activates neural reflexes regulating secretion in the guinea-pig colon. *Neurogastroenterol Motil* 1997; 9: 181-186.

[169] Kim M, Cooke HJ, Javed NH, Carey HV, Christofi F, Raybould HE. D-glucose releases 5-hydroxytryptamine from human BON cells as a model of enterochromaffin cells. *Gastroenterology* 2001; 121: 1400-1406.

[170] Gershon MD. Review article: serotonin receptors and transporters—roles in normal and abnormal gastrointestinal motility. *Aliment Pharmacol Ther* 2004; 20[Suppl 7]: 3-14.

[171] Bearcroft CP, Andre EA, Farthing MJ. In vivo effects of the 5-HT3 antagonist alosetron on basal and cholerat toxin-induced secretion in the human jejunum: a segmental perfusion study. *Aliment Pharmacol Ther* 1997; 11: 1109-1114.

[172] Ito M, Weber E, Hamel CT et al. Different expression of 5-HT4 receptor transcripts correlates with the functional responses of tegaserod on chloride/water secretion in the human ileum and colon in vitro. *Gastroenterology* 2006; 130: A544.

[173] Walsh JH. Gastrointestinal hormones. Johanson LR, Ed. Physiology of the gastrointestinal tract, 3rd ed. New York: Raven Press 1994.

[174] Spiller RC, Trotman IF, Higgins BE et al. The ileal brake - inhibition of jejunal motility after ileal fat perfusion in man. *Gut* 1984; 25: 365-374.

[175] Read NW, McFarlane A, Kinsman RI, Bates TE, Blackhall NW, Farrar GB, Hall JC, Moss G, Morris AP, O'Neill B, et al. Effect of infusion of nutrient solutions into the ileum on gastrointestinal transit and plasma levels of neurotensin and enteroglucagon. *Gastroenterology* 1984; 86: 274-280.

[176] Spiller RC, Jenkins D, Thornely Hebden JM, Wright T, Skinner M, Neal KR. |Increased rectal mucosal enteroendocrine cells, T lymphocytes, and increased gut permeability following acute Campylobacter enteritis and in post-dysenteric irritable bowel syndrome. *Gut* 2000; 47: 804-811.

[177] Dunlop SP, Jenkins D, Neal KR, Spiller RC. Relative importance of enterochromaffin cells hyperplasia, anxiety, and depression in postinfectious IBS. *Gastroenterology* 2003; 125: 1651-1659.

[178] Lee KJ, Kim YB, Kwon HC, Kim DK, Cho SW. The alteration of enterochromaffin cell, mast cell and lamnia propria T lymphocyte numbers in irritable bowel syndrome and its relationship with psychological factors. *J Gastroenterol Hepatol* 2008; 23: 1689-1694.

[179] Lee HS, Lim JH, Park H, Lee SI. Increased immunoreactive cells in intestinal mucosa of postinfectious irritable bowel syndrome patients 3 years after acute Shigella infection-an observation in a small case control study. *Yonsei Med J* 2009; 51: 45-51.

[180] Camilleri M. Is there a SERT-ain association with IBS. *Gut* 2004; 53: 1396-1398.

[181] Yeo A, Boyd P, Lumsden S, Saunders T, Handley A, Stubbins M, Knaggs A, Asquith S, Taylor I, Bahari B, Crocker N, Rallan R, Varsani S, Montgomery D, Alpers DH, Dukes GE, Purvis I, Hicks GA. Association between a functional polymorphism in the serotonin transporter gene and diarrhoea predominant irritable bowel syndrome in women. *Gut* 2004; 53: 1452-1458.

[182] Whorwell PJ, Clouter C, Smith CL. Oesophagus motility in the irritable bowel syndrome. *BMJ* 1981; 282: 1101-1102.

[183] Caballero-Plasencia AM, Valenzula-Barranco M, Herrerias-Gutierrez JM, Esteban-Carretero JM. Altered gastric emptying in patients with irritable bowel syndrome. *Eur Nul Med* 1999; 26: 404-409.

[184] Evans PR, Bak YT, Shuter B, Hoschl R, Kellow JE. Gastroparesis and small bowel dysmotility in irritable bowel syndrome. *Dig Dis Sci* 1997; 42: 2087-2093.

[185] van Wijk HJ, Smout AJ, Akkerman LM, Roelofs JM, ten Thije OJ. Gastric emptying and dyspeptic symptoms in irritable bowel syndrome. *Scand J Gastroenterol* 1992; 27: 99-102.

[186] Cann PA, Read NW, Brown C, Hobson N, Holdsworth CD. Irritable bowel syndrome: relation of disorders in the transit of single solid meal top symptom patterns. *Gut* 1983; 24: 405-411.

[187] Kellow JE, Philips SF. Altered small bowel motility in irritable bowel syndrome is correlated with symptoms. *Gastroenterology* 1987; 92: 1885-1893.

[188] Kellow JE, Philips SF, Miller LJ, Zinsmeister AR. Dysmotility of the small bowel in irritable bowel syndrome . *Gut* 1988; 29: 1236-1243.

[189] Mertz H, Naliboff B, Munakata J, Niazi N, Mayer EA. Altered rectal perception is a biological marker of patients with irritable bowel syndrome. *Gastroenterology* 1995; 109: 40-52.

[190] Lembo T, Munakata J, Mertz H, Niazi N, Kodner A, Nikas V, Mayer EA. Evidence for the hypersensitivity of lumbar splanchnic afferents in irritable bowel syndrome. *Gastroenterology* 1994; 107: 1686-1696.

[191] Munakata, Naliboff B, Harraf F, Kodner A, Lembo T, Chang L, Silverman DH, Mayer EA. Repetive sigmoid stimulation induces rectal hyperalgesia in patients with irritable bowel syndrome. *Gastroenterology* 1997; 112: 55-63.

[192] Van Ginkel R, Voskuijl WP, Benninga MA, Taminiau JA, Boeckxtaens GE. Alteration in rectal sensitivity and motility in childhood irritable bowel syndrome. *Gastroenterology* 2001; 120: 31-38.

[193] Verne GN, Robinson ME, Price DD. Hypersensitivity to visceral and coetaneous pain in irritable bowel syndrome. *Pain* 2001; 93: 7-14.

[194] Kanazawa M, Hongo M, Fukudo S. Viceral hypersensitivity in irritable bowel syndrome. *J Gastroenterol Hepatol* 2011; 26[Suppl 3]: 119-121.

[195] Nozu T, Okumura T. Viceral sensation and irritable bowel syndrome; with specia reference to comparison with functional abdominal syndrome. *J Gastroenterol Hepatol* 2011; 26[Suppl 3]: 122-127.

[196] El-Salhy M, Seim I, Chopin L, Gundersen D, Hatlebakk JG, Hausken T. Irritable bowel syndrome: the role of gut neuroendocrine peptides. *Front Biosci* 2012; E4: 2683-2700.

Chapter V

Post-Infectious and Inflammatory Bowel Disease Associated Irritable Bowel Syndrome

Abstract

Post-infectious IBS (PI-IBS) is defined as a sudden onset of IBS symptoms following gastroenteritis in individuals who previously have not any gastrointestinal complaints. This subset of IBS represents around 6% to 17% of patients with irritable bowel syndrome. Inflammatory bowel disease associated irritable bowel syndrome (IBD-IBS) is describing the occurrence of IBS symptoms in inflammatory disease (IBD) patients who are in remission. IBD-IBS occurs in 33 - 46% of ulcerative colitis patients, and in 42 - 60% of Crohn's disease patients in remission. Gastrointestinal infections, regardless of the pathogen, and probable non-gastrointestinal infection, cause PI-IBS in a considerable proportion of patients. The prevalence of PI-IBS decreases with time. It is possible that antibiotic treatment reduces the risk of developing PI-IBS, most likely by limiting the damage to the intestinal mucosa. This is an interesting aspect that needs to be explored further, as most gastroenteritis, which is self-limiting in nature, is not treated by antibiotics. Patients with both PI- and IBD-IBS exhibit low-grade mucosal inflammation and abnormalities in the neuroendocrine system of the gut. The main hormones affected in PI- and IBD-IBS, are small intestinal CCK, and large intestinal serotonin and PYY. The pathogenesis of these subsets of IBS fit well in our proposed hypothesis for the pathogenesis of IBS.

Introduction

The pathogenesis of IBS has been discussed in Chapter 4. Post-infectious and inflammatory bowel disease associated IBS (PI-IBS and IBD-IBS), is subset of IBS that constitute a considerable number of IBS patients, and their pathogenesis needs to be addressed at length. How the pathogenesis of this subset of IBS fits our hypothesis for IBS pathogenesis will be discussed further in this chapter.

5.1. Post-Infectious Irritable Bowel Syndrome (PI-IBS)

PI-IBS is defined as a sudden onset of IBS symptoms following gastroenteritis in individuals who previously have not any gastrointestinal complaints [1]. PI-IBS however, has also been reported following non-gastrointestinal infection such as respiratory, urinary tract and skin infections [2]. About 6% to 17% of patients with irritable bowel syndrome believe that their symptoms began with an infective illness [3]. Furthermore, between 7% and 31% of patients who suffer an acute episode of infectious gastroenteritis, develop PI-IBS despite clearance of the inciting pathogen [4]. Though acute gastroenteritis is common in the developing countries, the prevalence of IBS in the population is lower than in the developed countries [4-9]. It has been speculated that this may be caused by modulation of the immune system to a Th2 type response (caused by other infection such as with helminthes), a higher degree of tolerance by the host (caused by exposure to these infections from early childhood) and host genetic factors [5, 10]. The low prevalence of IBS in the developing countries can also be attributed to racial and cultural difference in health-care-seeking behaviour. Thus, Hispanics and Asians are less likely than Caucasians to seek health-care for bowel complaints, and Hispanics are also more likely to self-medicate with folk remedies to maintain good bowel function [8, 11].

The clinical phenomenon of PI-IBS was first described more than six decades ago by Stewart, who coined the term "postdysenteric colitis", to describe continued symptoms of diarrhoea in British troops after successful treatment of amoebic dysentery [12]. He declared that a primary attack of dysentery may be followed by a chronic disorder of the colon. He stated further, that in amoebiasis this disorder is more common than in bacillary infection, and that only a small proportion of patients suffered from this disorder [12]. More than a decade ago, Chaudhary and Truelove described 34 patients, out of 130 cases who had bowel symptoms after an attack of bacillary or amoebic dysentery, and they coined the term "postdysenteric irritable bowel syndrome" [13]. In south India, 10% of subjects in a rural community who experienced an attack of gastroenteritis, continued to have increased frequency and liquidity of the stool [14]. This was described as post-infective malabsorption syndrome, though only a small proportion of these individuals were tested and shown to have malabsorption [15-17]. These observations did not receive the immediate attention they deserved. It was not until over 30 years later that another publication sparked wider interest in the development of IBS, after an acute episode of infectious gastroenteritis [18].

The incidence and natural history of PI-IBS has now been more fully investigated, following a large outbreak of acute gastroenteritis caused by food-borne norovirus at the annual meeting of the Canadian Society of Gastroenterology [19]. After three months, 23.6% reported symptoms consistent with PI-IBS. At six, 12 and 24 months, the prevalence of IBS was similar among those exposed, versus non-exposed individuals [19]. Thus, PI-IBS is common after viral gastroenteritis, but it seems to be transient. It is noteworthy that a study of 243 subjects who suffered an acute episode of infectious mononucleosis, a non-gastrointestinal viral infection, revealed that 7% developed PI-IBS at three months, and 8% at six months, following the infection [20].

Human infections caused by *Campylobacter jejuni* are a leading cause of foodborne enteritis, usually transmitted by the ingestion of undercooked poultry, or contact with farm animals, and accounts for 10% of gastroenteritis in England and Wales [21-23]. *Campylobacter jejuni* produces a range of toxins including cytolethal distending toxin [24], which first produces secretory diarrhoea in the small intestine early in the illness, after which there is invasion of the distal ileum and colon to produce an inflammatory ileocolitis, which can extend all the way to the rectum [25]. In a prospective study of 592 patients with an acute episode of *Campylobacter* gastroenteritis, 15% had developed IP-IBS at three months and 11% at six months following the infection [20]. In another prospective study, including 620 patients suffering from *Campylobacter* gastroenteritis, the incidence of PI-IBS amounted to 15% and 10% at three and six month follow-up, respectively [26]. In another study, PI-IBS following *Campylobacter* gastroenteritis was been found to be 13.8% [5, 27]. Gastroenteritis caused by *Salmonella spp.* accounted for 3% of all cases in England and Wales [23]. Following gastroenteritis caused by *Salmonella spp.*, between 11.6% of 677, and 31% of 38 patients, developed PI-IBS after 12 months [18, 28]. Twelve months post *Shigella* infection 10.5% of the patients developed PI-IBS [29]. In another study, 14.9% of the patients who had *Shigella* infection, had developed PI-IBS at the three year follow-up [30]. Two years following *Shigella* infection in 295 patients, 8.1% had developed PI-IBS [31]. It seems however, that patients with PI-IBS following infection recover after five years [32]. *Clostridium difficile* infection is responsible for almost all cases of pseudomembranous colitis [33], and for about 20% of cases of antibiotic-associated diarrhoea without colitis [34, 35]. In a separate study, only one patient of 23 infected with *Clostridium difficile* had developed PI-IBS three months after the infection (4.3%) [36]. This result is rather surprising, as it is an aggressive bacteria that is known to cause extensive damage to the intestinal mucosa. It is noteworthy however, that all patients included in this study received metronidazole for seven days, and bacteriological examinations were repeated at the end of treatment to ensure the absence of infection. Is it possible therefore that the antibiotic treatment affected the outcome? In a rat model of PI-IBS, after *Campylobacter* infection, prophylactic treatment with rifaximin mitigated the development of IBS [37].

In 2000, a large waterborne outbreak of bacterial dysentery occurred at Walkerton in Ontario, Canada. The pathogens behind this dysentery were identified as *Escherichia coli* 0157:H7 and *Campylobacter jejuni.* A total of 4,561 individuals were included in a follow up study [38, 39]. The incidence of PI-IBS was 28.6% two to three years following the gastroenteritis [38]. This incidence declined to 21.4% at four years, 14.3% at six years and 15.4% at eight years [39]. Instability of the PI-IBS subtypes over time was observed [39], and this instability is similar to that observed in sporadic (unselected) IBS [40]. In 189 patients with an intestinal bacterial infection caused by *Salmonella* (52%) and *Campylobacter* (42%), nearly 10% reported PI-IBS up to 10 years later [41].

PI-IBS incidence was been found to be 3.7%, three months post acute enteric infection in a prospective cohort study of 118 patients, recruited from three health regions in Ontario, Canada [42]. The enteric pathogens in these patients were *Campylobacter* (51.5%), *Gardia lambila* (21.6%), *Salmonella* (16.9%), *Entamoeba histolytica* (1.3%), *E. coli* (4.3%), *Yersinia* (2.6%) and

Shigella (1.7%). In the Netherlands, 9% of patients with bacterial gastroenteritis caused by *Campylobacter, Salmonella* or *Shigella* developed IBS two years after infection [43]. A cohort of 318 patients who had acute gastroenteritis caused by *Campylobacter* (54%), *Salmonella* (37%) and other organisms (9%), and 584 308 subjects without history of IBS from the background population were followed-up for a year [44]. Six months after bacterial gastroenteritis, 6.3% of patients developed PI-IBS [43]. About 40% of the patients, however, recovered after six years [45]. Interestingly, 44% of patients with sporadic IBS had also been found to recover after six years when followed-up [45]. PI-IBS developed in 29% of 75 patients, three months after they had suffered acute gastroenteritis [46]. Three months following an acute gastroenteritis, 23% out of 94 patients exhibited PI-IBS [47]. At 12 month follow-up, only 13% of these patients still had PI-IBS [48].

Traveller's diarrhoea is an acute infectious disease that is responsive to antibiotic therapy and is self-limited in nature. The microbial pathogens most likely to be isolated in persistent traveller's diarrhoea are protozoans [49]. *Giardia spp.* are the most common protozoan pathogen in returned travellers. Other protozoans such as *Cyclospora, Cryptosporidium spp., Dientamoeba fragilis* and *Entamoeba histolytica* can also be pathogens responsible for traveller's diarrhoea [49]. Six months after gastroenteritis, mostly due to *E. coli*, acquired during a five week stay in Mexico, 10% out of 61 North American patients developed PI-IBS [50]. In another study, on travellers from Canada and the USA, it was revealed that 4.2% develop PI-IBS three months following acute gastroenteritis [51]. PI-IBS developed in 13.6% out of 118 patients six month after an acute gastroenteritis acquired during travelling in Asia (84%), and in both South Africa and South America (5%) [52].

In 2004, an extensive outbreak of waterborne giardiasis occurred in Bergen, Norway, where 1,300 cases were confirmed to have *Giardia* by stool examination [53]. The Norwegian Prescription Database gave an estimate of 2,500 cases treated for giardiasis probably linked to the outbreak [53]. Twelve to thirty months after the onset of *Giardia* infection, 80.5% out of 82 patients exhibited PI-IBS [54], and showed increased visceral sensitivity [55]. The high incidence of gastrointestinal symptoms observed after *Giardia* infection, can be explained by the finding that 32.3% out of 124 patients, over the 15 month period post *Giardia* infection, suffered from chronic *Giardia* infection [56].

In 2003 - 2004 a large outbreak of trichinellosis, caused by the nematode *Trichinella britovi*, occurred in Izmir, Turkey. Seventy-two patients with trichinellosis, but without pre-existing IBS, and 27 uninfected subjects were followed-up two, four, six and 12 months after infection [57]. Six and 12 months following trichinellosis, 13.9% and 7% exhibited PI-IBS, respectively [57]. None of the uninfected subjects showed any signs of IBS during the observation time.

From the data presented above, it is clear that gastrointestinal infections, regardless of the pathogen, and also probably non-gastrointestinal infection, cause PI-IBS in a considerable proportion of patients. The prevalence of PI-IBS decreases with time and is possible that antibiotic treatment reduces the development of PI-IBS, most likely by limiting the damage to the intestinal mucosa. This is an interesting aspect that needs to be explored further, as most gastroenteritis, which is self-limited in nature, is not treated by antibiotics.

5.1.1. Risk factors for developing of PI-IBS

The risk for developing PI-IBS can be divided into host related risk factors, and the infecting-organism associated risk factors. This subject has been presented and discussed in a number of recent reviews, which the reader is referred to [4, 23, 58-62].

5.1.2. Low-Grade Inflammation in PI-IBS

The intestinal mucosa of patients with PI-IBS, as well as in animal models of PI-IBS, shows a low-grade inflammation. Thus, in patients with chronic giardiasis (patients with *Giardia* infection despite antibiotic treatment), as well as in patients with PI-IBS following *Giardia* infection, an increased intraepithelial infiltration of lymphocytes has been observed in the duodenal mucosa [63] (Figures 23 and 24). The lymphocyte infiltration in chronic giardiasis was much more prominent than in PI-IBS [63]. Similarly, an increased infiltration of T lymphocytes, as well as mast cells, has been reported in the duodenal and jejunal mucosa of an animal model for PI-IBS [64]. In the terminal ileum of PI-IBS patients following Shigella infection, an increase in the number of mast cells has also been seen [31]. Furthermore, an increase in the expression of Il-m RNA has been found in the ilial and colonic mucosa of the same patients [31].

The density of T lymphocytes and mast cells was increased in the lamina propria of the rectum in patients with PI-IBS [65, 66]. Similarly, serial rectal biopsies taken from patients following *Campylobacter* enteritis, showed an increase in the density of CD3, CD4 and CD8 lymphocytes, both intraepithelial and in the lamina propria [67]. This increase persisted for more than a year after infection [67].

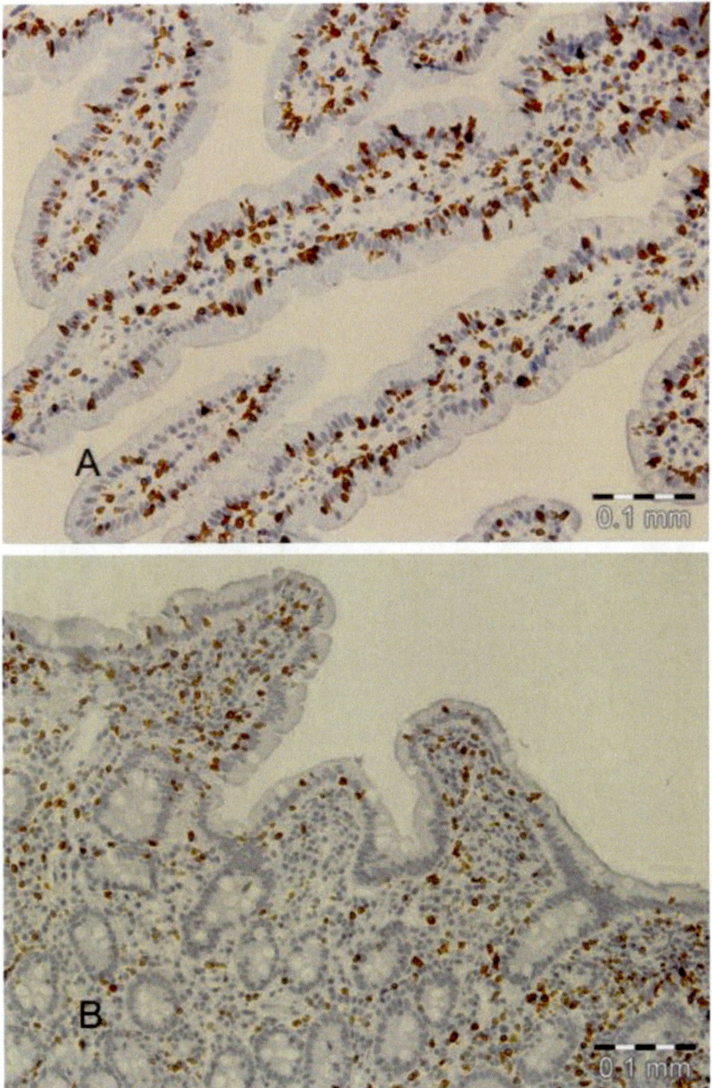

These photomicrographs are provided kindly by Dr. Vernesa Dizdar, Section of Gastroenterology, Institute of Medicine, Bergen University, Norway.

Figure 23. CD3 lymphocyte infiltration in a healthy subject (A), and in a patient with chronic giardiasis (B).

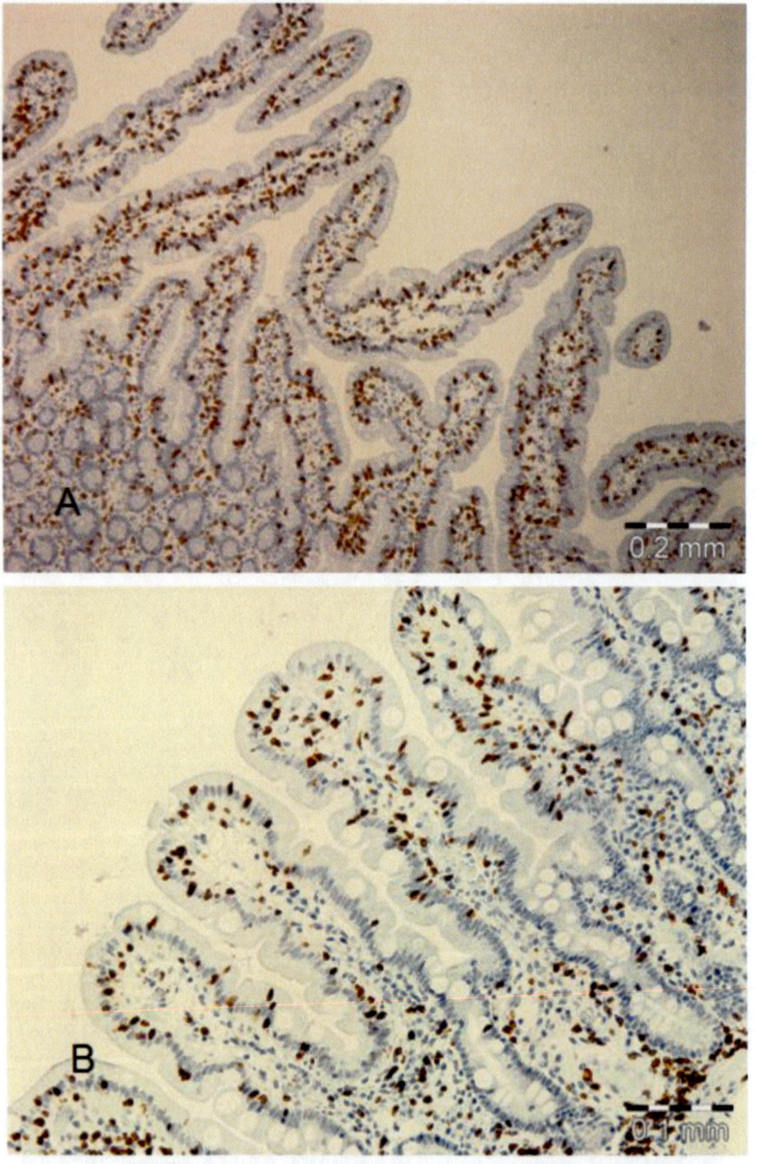

These photomicrographs are provided kindly by Dr. Vernesa Dizdar, Section of Gastroenterology, Institute of Medicine, Bergen University, Norway.

Figure 24. The infiltration CD3 lymphocytes in a healthy subject (A), and in a patient with PI-IBS following *Giardia* infection (B).

5.1.3. Abnormality in the Neuroendocrine System of the Gut in PI-IBS

Several abnormalities in the neuroendocrine system (NES) of the gut have been reported in patients with PI-IBS following infections with different pathogens and in experimental animals (see Table 6).

Table 6. Overview of the abnormalities in the neuroendocrine system of the gut in sporadic-, PI- and IBD-IBS

	IBS	PI-IBS	IBD-IBS
Stomach **Ghrelin**	**High IBS-D** **Low IBS-C**	**?**	**?**
Small Intestine CCK	Low	High	?
Secretin	Low	?	?
GIP	Low	?	?
Somatostatin	Low	?	Low
Serotonin	Unchanged	High	Low
Large intestine Serotonin	Low	High	High/low
PYY	Low	High	Low
PP	?	?	Low
Entroglucagon	?	?	High

In the small intestine, duodenal CCK and serotonin cell densities were increased in PI-patients following giardiasis [68]. Furthermore, plasma CCK increased postprandially in these patients [68]. In a mouse model of PI-IBS, duodenal and jejunal serotonin cell densities were also increased [63]. Moreover, serotonin transporter (SERT) expression was decreased in this animal model [63].

In the large intestine, serotonin cell density was increased in PI-IBS, regardless of the pathogen [31, 65-67, 69]. Moreover, high plasma level of serotonin has been reported to occur in PI-IBS postprandially [70]. Furthermore, high PYY cell density has been observed in PI-IBS patients following acute *Shigella* infection [31].

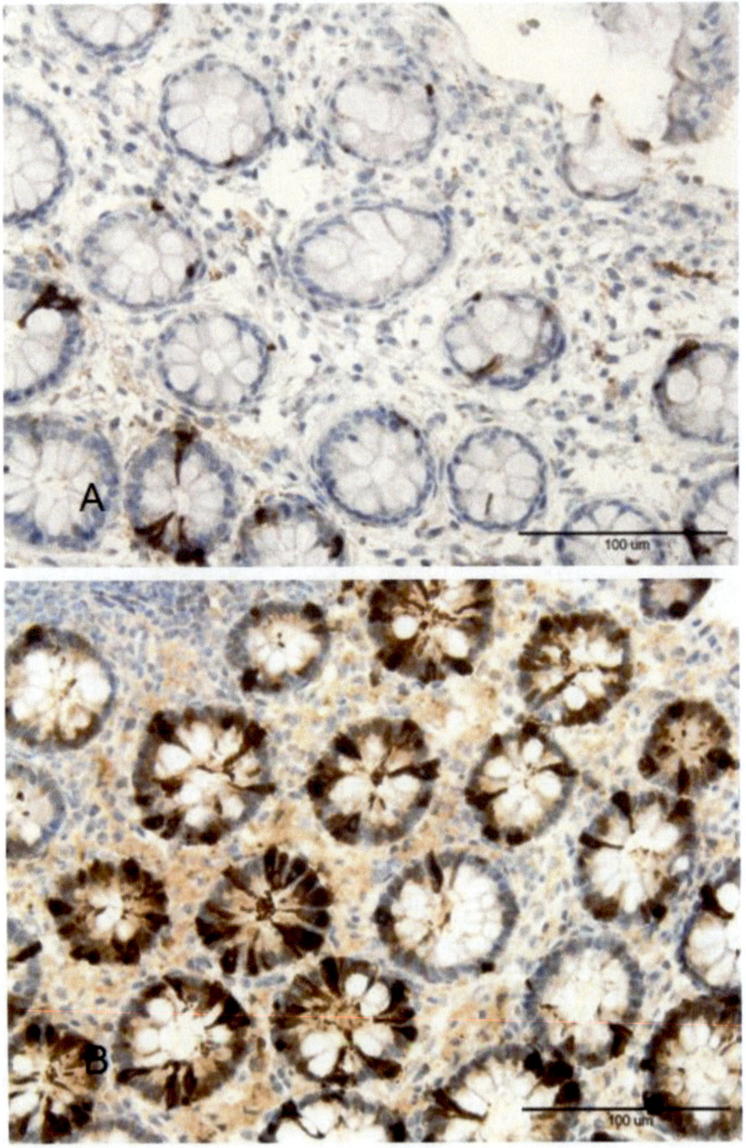

Figure 25. Serotonin immunoreactive cells in the colon of a control who underwent colonoscopy due to rectal bleeding and the cause of bleeding was found to be haemorrhoids (A), and in the colon of a patient with ulcerative colitis (B).

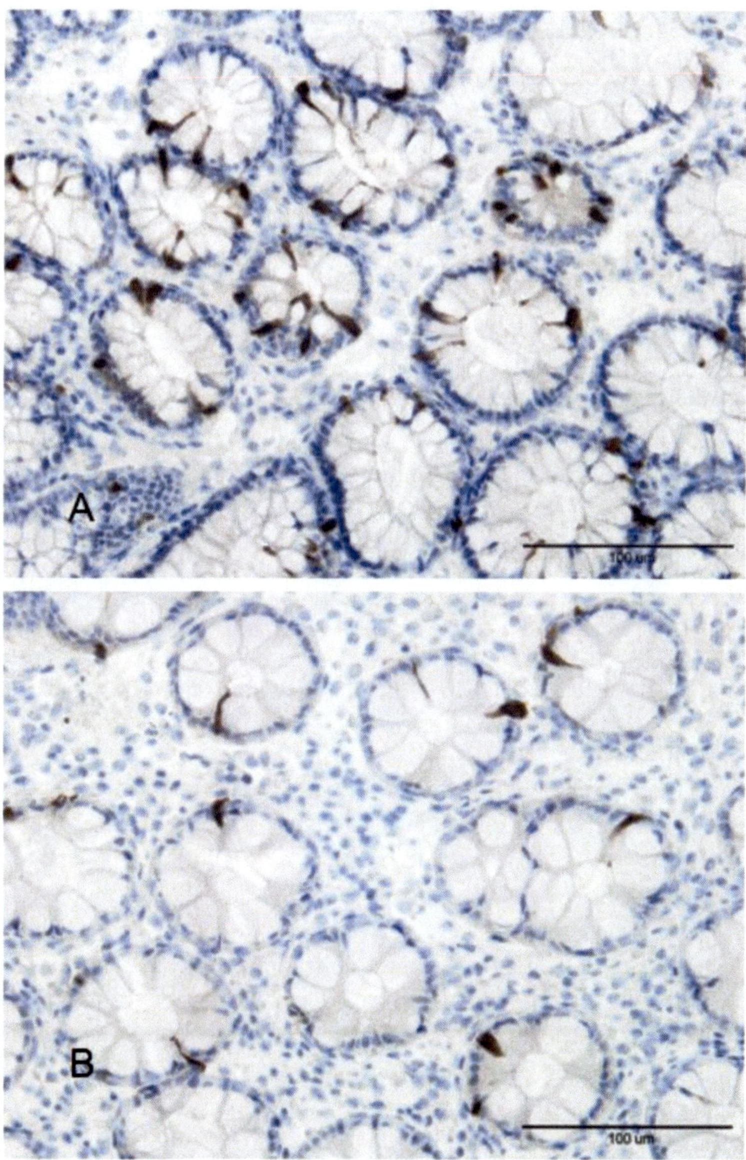

Figure 26. Enteroglucagon immunoreactive cells in a control who underwent colonoscopy due to health concerns caused by a relatives being diagnosed with colon carcinoma (A), and in the colon of a patient with Crohn's disease (B).

5.2. Inflammatory Bowel Disease Associated Irritable Bowel Syndrome (IA-IBS)

Inflammatory bowel diseases (IBD) comprise ulcerative colitis (UC) and Crohn's disease (CD). These diseases are chronic and their clinical courses differs considerably, with frequent relapses or chronic active disease in some patients, whereas some have years of virtually complete remission (71). Clinicians are often challenged to interpret gastrointestinal symptoms in patients with IBD in remission. IBS was found in 33% of 98 patients, and in 46% of 50 patients, with UC in remission [72, 73]. Other studies have shown that IBS occurs in 32 - 39% of UC patients, and in 42 - 60% of CD patients in remission [74-76]. Faecal calprotectin has been found to be significantly elevated in UC and CD patients with criteria for IBS, compared to those without IBS-type symptoms, indicating the presence of occult inflammation [76].

5.2.1. Abnormalities in the Neuroendocrine System of the Gut in IBD

About fifteen years ago, El-Salhy and colleges demonstrated that colonic serotonin and enteroglucagon immunoreactivity was elevated in patients with UC and CD [77]. Whereas, areas of peptide YY (PYY) and pancreatic poly-peptide were decreased [77]. As enteroglucagon and PYY are colocalised in the same colorectal endocrine cell type (L-cells) [78-81], it seems that this cell increased the expression of enteroglucagon, and reduced the expression of PYY. In one study, serotonin cell density in rectal biopsies from patients with UC was found to be elevated [82], whereas another study showed it to be decreased [83]. In rectal biopsies from patients with UC mucosal serotonin, tryptophan hydroxylase 1 messenger RNA, serotonin transporter messenger and serotonin transporter were all reduced [83]. In the ileum mucosa of patients with CD, the cell densities of serotonin, somatostatin, PP and PYY are decreased [84]. Fasting plasma level and rectal tissue extracts from patients with UC have also been reported to be reduced [85].

In an experimental animal model of colitis (IL2 knockout mice), serotonin and PYY cell densities decreased in mice with colitis, whereas enteroglucagon was unchanged [86]. In another animal model (rats treated with dextran sulfate sodium), the PYY concentration decreased in the small and large intestine [87]. As regard to substance P (SP) and vasoactive intestinal polypeptide (VIP), controversial results have been reported both in patients with UC and CD, and experimental animal models, as to whether they increase or decrease during inflammation [82, 84, 86, 88-90].

5.3. The Pathogenesis of PI- and IBD-IBS

There is convincing evidence that patients with PI-IBS and IBD-IBS have low-grade inflammation. It is noteworthy that 50% of IBS patients have been reported to have a significant infiltration of immunocytes [91]. This high percentage raises the question as to whether half of IBS patients suffer from either PI- or IBD-IBS? This low grade inflammation can cause changes in the neuroendocrine system of the gut, as discussed earlier in Chapter 4. Abnormalities in the neuroendocrine system of the gut have been observed in PI- and IBD-IBS patients. The three main gut hormones that seem to be involved in IBS are CCK, serotonin and PYY (see Table 6). The nature of abnormalities is different between sporadic IBS on one hand, and PI- and IBD-IBS on the other. The pathogenesis of PI- and IBD-IBS, therefore fits well in the hypothesis proposed earlier (see Chapter 4).

A question that arises is: why do only a proportion of patients that suffer gastroenteritis, or are affected by IBD, developed low grade inflammation? Genetic factors can be of importance, as an association of the *TNFSF15* polymorphism with irritable bowel syndrome has been reported [92]. *TNFSF15* gene is involved in the regulation of immune and inflammatory responses.

References

[1]   Ghoshal UC, Park H, Gwee KA. Bugs and irritable bowel syndrome: the good, the bad and the ugly. *J Gastroenterol Hepatol* 2010; 25:244-251.

[2]   Mckeown ES, Parry D, Stansfield JR, Barton R, Welfare MR. Postinfectious irritable bowel syndrome may occur after non-gastrointestinal and intestinal infection. *Neurogastroenterol Motil* 1006; 18: 839-843.

[3]   Longstreth CF, Hawkey CJ, Mayer EA, Jones RH, Naesdal J, Wilson IK, Peacock RA, Wiklund IK. Characteristics of patients with irritable bowel syndrome recruited from three sources: implications for clinical trials. *Allment Pharmacol Ther* 2001; 15: 959-964.

[4]   Spiller R, Garsed. Infection, inflammation and the irritable bowel syndrome. *Dig Liver Dis* 2009; 41: 844-840.

[5]   Ghoshal U, Ranjan P. Post-infectious irritable bowel syndrome: the past, the present and the future. *J Gastroenterol Hepatol* 2011; 26 (Suppl 3): 94-101.

[6]   Ghoshal UC, Abraham P, Bhatt C, Choudhuri G, Bhatia SJ, Shenoy KT, Banka NH, Bose K, Bohidar NP, Chakravartty K, Shekhar NC, Desai N, Dutta U, Das G, Dutta S, Dixit VK, Goswami BD, Jain RK, Jain S, Jayanthi V, Kochhar R, Kumar A, Makharia G, Mukewar SV, Mohan Prasad VG, Mohanty A, Mohan AT, Sathyaprakash BS, Prabhakar B, Philip M, Veerraju EP, Ray G, Rai RR, Seth AK, Sachdeva A, Singh SP, Sood A, Thomas V, Tiwari S, Tandan M, Upadhyay R, Vij JC. Epidemiological and clinical profile of irritable bowel syndrome in India: report of the Indian society of gastroenterology task force. *Indian J Gastroenterol* 2008; 27: 22-28.

[7]   Danivar D, Tankeyoon M, Sriratanaban A. Prevalence of irritable bowel syndrome in a non-Western population. *Br Med J* (Clin Res Ed) 1988; 296:1710.

[8]   Masud MA, Hasan M, Khan AK. Irritable bowel syndrome in a rural community in Bangladesh: prevalence, symptoms pattern, and health care seeking behavior . *Am J Gastroenterol* 2001; 96: 1547-1552.

[9]   Husain N, Chaudhry IB, Jafri F, Niaz SK, Tomenson B, Creed FA. Population-based study of irritable bowel syndrome in non-Western population. *Neurogastroenterol Motil* 2008; 20: 1022-1029.

[10]   Pearce EJ, Kane C, Sun J, Taylor J, Mckee AS, Cervi L. Th2 response polarization during infection with the helminth parasite Schistosoma mansoni. *Immunol Rev* 2004; 20: 117-126.

[11]   Zuckerman MJ,Guerra LG, Drossman DA, Foland JA, Gregory GG. Health-care-seeking behaviors related to bowel complains. Hispanics versus non-Hispanic whites. *Dig Dis Sci* 1996; 41: 77-82.

[12]   Stewart GT. Post-dysenteric colitis. *BJM* 1950; 1: 405-409.

[13]   Chaudhary NA, Truelove SC. The irritable colon syndrome. A study of the clinical features, predisposing causes and prognosis in 130 cases. *Q J Med* 1962; 31: 307-322.

[14] Mathan VI, Baker SJ. Epidemic tropical sprue and other epidemics of diarrhea in South Indian villages. *Am J Clin Nutr* 1968; 21: 1077-1087.

[15] Montgomery RD, Shearer AC. The cell population of the upper jejunal mucosa in tropic sprue and postinfective malabsorption. *Gut* 1974; 15: 387-391.

[16] Lindenbaum J. malabsorption during and after recovery from acute intestinal infection. *Br Med J* 1965; 2: 326-329.

[17] Ramakrishna BS, Venkataraman S, Mukhopadhya A. Tropical malabsorption. *Postgrad Med* J 2006: 82: 779-787.

[18] McKendrick MW, Read NW. Irritable bowel syndrome -post salmonella infection. *J Infect* 1994; 29: 1-3.

[19] Marshall JK, Thabane M, Borgaonkar MR, James C. Postinfectious irritable bowel syndrome after a food-borne outbreak of acute gastroenteritis attributed to a viral pathogen. can *Gastroenterol Hepatol* 2007; 5: 457-460.

[20] Moss-Morris R, Spence M. To "lump" or to "split" the functional somatic syndromes: can infectious and emotional risk factors differentiate between the onset of chronic fatigue syndrome and irritable bowel syndrome. *Psychosom Med* 2006; 68: 463-469.

[21] Friedman CR, Hoekstra RM, Samul, Marcus R, Bender J, Shiferaw B, Reddy S, Ahuja SD, Helfrick DL, Hardnett F, Carter M, Anderson B, Tauxe RV, Emerging Infections Program FoodNet Working Group. Risk factors for sporadic Campylobacter infection in the united States: a case-control study in Food-Net sites. *Clin Infect Dis* 2004; 38 Suppl 3): S285-S296.

[22] Kapperud G, Skjerve E, Bean NH, Ostroff SM, Lassen J. Risk factors for sporadic Campylobacter infections: results of a case-control study in southeastern Norway. *J Clin Microbiol* 1992; 30: 3117-3121.

[23] Spiller R, Garsed K. Postinfectious irritable bowel syndrome. *Gastroenterology* 2009; 136: 1979-1988.

[24] Whitehouse CA, Bablo PB, Prsci EC, Cottle DL, Mirabito PM, Pickett CL. *Campylobacter jejuni* cytolethal distending toxin causes a G2-phase cell cycle block. Infect Immun 1998; 66: 1934-1940.

[25] Rutgeerts P, Geboes K, Ponette E, Coremans G, Vantrappen G. Acute infective colitis caused by endemic pathogens in Western Europe. Endoscopic features. *Endoscopy* 1982; 14: 212-219.

[26] Spence M, Moss-Morris R. The cognitive behavioural model of irritable bowel syndrome: a prospective investigation of patients with gastroenteritis. *Gut* 2007; 56: 1066-1071.

[27] Dunlop SP, Jenkins D, Spiller RC. Distinctive clinical, psychological, and histological features of postinfective irritable bowel syndrome. *Am J Gastroenterol* 2003; 98: 1578-1583.

[28] Mearin F, Pèrez-Oliveras M, Perellò A, Vinyet J, Ibannñez A, Coderch J, Perona M. Dyspepsia and irritable bowel syndrome after a salmonella gastroenteritis outbreak: one-year follow-up cohort study. *Gastroenterology* 2005; 129: 98-104.

[29] Ji S, Park H, Lee D, Song YK, Choi JP, Lee SI. Post-infectious irritable bowel syndrome in patients with Shigella infection. *J Gastroenterol Hepatol* 2005; 20:381-386.

[30] Kim HS, Kim Ms, Ji SW, Park H. The development of irritable bowel syndrome after Shigella infection: 3 year follow-up study. *Korean J Gastroenterol* 2006; 47: 300-305.

[31] Wang L-H, Fang X-C, Pan G-Z. Bacillary dysentery as a causative factor for irritable bowel syndrome and its pathogenesis. *Gut* 2004; 53: 1096-1101.

[32] Jung IS, Kim HS, Park H, Lee SI. The clinical course of postinfectious irritable bowel syndrome: a five-year follow-up study. *J Clin Gastroenterol* 2009; 43:534-540.

[33] Hurley BW, Nguen CC. The spectrum of pseudomembranous entrocolitis and antibiotic-associated diarrhea. *Arch Intern Med* 2002; 162: 2177-2184.

[34] Dalla RM, Harbrecht BG, Boujoukas AJ, Sirio CA, Farkas LM, Lee KK, Simmons RL. Fulminant *Clostridium difficile:* An unappreciated and increasing cause of death and complications:*Ann Surg* 2002: 235: 363-372.

[35] Kyne L, Hamel MB, Polavaram R, Kelly CP. Health care costs and mortality with nosocomial diarrhea due to *Clostridium difficile. Clin Infect Dis* 2002; 34: 346-353.

[36] Piche T, Vanbiervliet, Pipau FG, Dainese R, Hèbuterne X, Rampal P, Collins SM. Low risk of irritable bowel syndrome *Clostridium difficile* after infection. *Can J Gastroenterol* 2007; 21: 727-731.

[37] Pimentel M, Morales W, Jee S-R, Low K, Hwang L, Pokkunuri V, Micocha J, Conklin J, Chang C. Antibiotic prophylaxis prevents the development of post-infectious phenotype in a new rat model of post-infectious IBS. *Dig Dis Sci* 2011; 56: 1962-1966.

[38] Marshall JK, Thabane M, Garg AX, Clark WF, Salvadori M, Collins SM, The Walkerton health study investigators. Incidence and

epidemiology of irritable bowel syndrome after a large waterborne outbreak of bacterial dysentery. *Gastroenterology* 2006; 131:445-450.

[39] Marshall JK, Thabane M, Garg AX, Clark WF, Moayyedi P, Collins SM, The Walkerton health study investigators. Eight years prognosis of postinfectious irritable bowel syndrome following waterborne bacterial dysentery. *Gut* 2010; 59:605-611.

[40] Engsbro AL, Simrèn M, Bytzer P. Short-term stability of subtypes in the irritable bowel syndrome: prospective evaluation using Rome III classification. *Aliment Pharmacol Ther* 2011; doi:10.1111/j.1365-2036.2011.04948.x.

[41] Schwille-Kiuntke J, Enck P, Zendler C, Krieg M, Polster AV, Klosterhalfen S, Autenerieth IB, Zipfel S, Frick JS. Postinfectious irritable bowel syndrome: follow-up of a patient cohort of confirmed cases of bacterial infection with Salmonella or Campylobacter. *Neurogastroenterol Motil* 2011; 23: e479-e488.

[42] Borgaonkar MR, Ford DC, Marshall JK, Churchill E, Collins SM. The incidence of irritable bowel syndrome among community subjects with previous acute enteric infection. *Dig Dis Sci* 2006; 51: 1026-1032.

[43] Haagsma JA, Siersema PD, De Wit NJ, Havelaar AH. Disease burden of post-infectious irritable bowel syndrome in the Netherlands. *Epidemiol Infect* 2010; 138: 1650-156.

[44] Rodriguez LAC, Ruigòmez A. Increased risk of irritable bowel syndrome after bacterial gastroenteritis: cohort study. *BMJ* 1999; 318: 565-566.

[45] Neal KR, Hebden J, Spiller R. Prevalence of gastrointestinal symptoms six months after bacterial gastroenteritis and risk factors for development of the irritable bowel syndrome: postal survey of patients. *BMJ* 1997; 314: 779-782.

[46] Neal KR, Barker L, Spiller R. Prognosis in post-infective irritable bowel syndrome: a six year follow up study. *Gut* 2002; 51: 410-413.

[47] Gwee KA, Graham JC, Mckendrick MW, Collins SM, Marshall JS, Walters SJ, Read NW. Psychometric scores and persistence of irritable bowel after infectious diarrhoea. *Lancet* 1996; 347: 150-153.

[48] Gwee KA, Leong YL, Graham C, Mckendrick MW, Collins SM, Walters SJ, Underwood JE, Read NW. The role of psychological and biological factors in postinfective gut dysfunction. *Gut* 1999; 44: 400-406.

[49] Connor BA. Sequelae of traveller's diarrhea: focus on postinfectiuos irritable bowel syndrome. *Clin Infect Dis* 2005; 41: S577-S586.

[50] Okhuysen PC, Jiang ZD, Carlin L, Forbes C, DuPont HL. Post-diarrhea chronic intestinal symptoms and irritable bowel syndrome in North American travelers to Mexico. *Am J Gastroenterol* 2004; 99: 1774-1778.

[51] Ilnyckyi A, Balachandra S, Elliott L, Choudhri S, Duerksen DR. Post-traveler's diarrhea irritable bowel syndrome: a prospective study. *Am J Gastroenterol* 2003; 98: 596-599.

[52] Stermer E, Lubezky A, Potaman I, Paster E, Lavy A. Is traveler's diarrhea a significant risk factor for the development of irritable bowel syndrome? A prospective study. *Clin Infect Dis* 2006; 43: 898-901.

[53] Nygård K, Schimmer B, Sobstad Ø, Walde A, Tveit I, Langeland N, Hausken T, Aavitsland P. A large community outbreak of waterborne giardiasis-delayed detection in non-endemic urbane area. *BMC Public Health* 2006; 6: 141-151.

[54] Hanevik K, Dizdar, Langeland N, Hausken T. Development of functional gastrointestinal diorders after *Giardia lambia* infection. *BMC Gastroenterol* 2009; 9: 27-31.

[55] Dizdar V, Gilja OH, Hausken T. Increased visceral sensitivity in *Giardia*-induced postinfectious irritable bowel syndrome and functional dyspepsia. Effect of the 5HT3-antagonist ondansetron. *Neurogastroenterol Motil* 2007; 19: 977-982.

[56] Hanevik K, Hausken T, Morken MH, Strand EA, Mørch K, Coll P, Helgeland L, Langeland N. Persisting symptoms and duodenal inflammation related to *Giardia duodenalis* infection. *J infect* 2007; 55: 524-530.

[57] Soyturk M, Akpinar H, Gurler O, Pozio E, Sari I, Akar S, Akarsu M, Birlik M, Onen F, Akkoc N. Irritable bowel syndrome in persons who acquired trichinellosis. Am J Gastroenterol 2007; 102: 1064-1069.

[58] Spiller CR. Role of infection in irritable bowel syndrome. *J Gastroenterology* 2007; 42: 41-47.

[59] Sarna SK. Lessons learnt from post-infectious IBS. Front Physiol 2011; 2: 1-13. doi:10.3389/fphys.2011.00049.

[60] Gwee K-A. Post-infectious irritable bowel syndrome, an inflammation-immunological model with relevance for other IBS and functional dyspepsia. *J Neurogastroenterol Motil* 2010; 16: 30-34.

[61] Halvorson HA, Schlett CD, Riddle MS. Postinfectious irritable bowel syndrome -a meta-analysis. *Am J Gastroenterol* 2006; 101: 1894-1899.

[62] Spiller R. Serotonin, inflammation, and IBS: Fitting the jigsaw together. *J Pediatr Gastroenterol Nutr* 2007; 45: S115-S119.

[63] Dizdar V, Hanevik K, Lærum OD, Gilja OH, Langeland N, Hausken T. Duodenal mucosal lymphocytes in giardia-induced functional gastrointestinal disorder. Abstract presented at the 19th United European Gastroenterology Week (UEGW) 2011.

[64] Wheatcorf J, Wakekin D, Smith A, Mahoney R, Mawe G, Spiller R. Enterochromaffin cell hyperplasia and decreased serotonin transporter in a mouse model of postinfectious bowel dysfunction. *Neurogastroenterol Motil* 2005; 17: 863-870.

[65] Dunlop SP, Jenkins D, Spiller RC. Distinctive clinical, psychological and histological feature of postinfective irritable bowel syndrome. *Am J Gastroenterol* 2003; 98: 1578-1583.

[66] Lee KJ, Kim YB, Kim JH, Kwon HC, Kim DK, Cho SW. The alteration of enterochromaffin cell, mast cell and lamina propria T lymphocytes number s in irritable bowel syndrome and its relation with psychological factors. *J Gastroenterol Hepatol* 2008; 23: 1689.1694.

[67] Spiller RC, Jenkins D, Thornley JP, Hebden JM, Wright T, Skinner M, Neal KR. Increased rectal mucosal enterochromaffin cells, T lymphocytes, and increased gut permeability following acute Campylobacter enteritis and in post-dysenteric irritable bowel syndrome. *Gut* 2000; 47; 804-811.

[68] Dizdar V, Spiller R, Hanevik K, Gilja OH, El-Salhy M, Hausken T. Relative importance of CCK (cholecystokinin) and 5-HT (serotonin) in Giardia-induced Post-infectious IBS. *Aliment Pharmacol Ther* 2010; 31: 883-891.

[69] Kim HS, Lim JH, Park H, Lee SI. Increased immunoendocrine cells in intestinal mucosa of postinfectious irritable bowel syndrome patients 3 years after acute *Shigella* infection- an observation in small case control study. *Yonsei Med J* 2010; 51: 45-51.

[70] Dunlop SP, Coleman NS, Blackshow E, Perkins AC, Singh G, Marsden CA, Spiller RC. Abnormalities of 5-hydroxytryptamine metabolism in irritable bowel syndrome. *Clin Gastroenterol Hepatol* 2005; 3: 349-357.

[71] Andres PG, Friedman LS. Epidemiology and natural course of inflammatory bowel disease. *Gastroenterol Clin North Am* 1999; 28: 255-281.

[72] Isgar B, Harman M, Kaye MD, Whorwell PJ. Symptoms of irritable bowel syndrome in ulcerative colitis remission. *Gut* 1983; 24; 190-192.

[73] Ansari R, Attari F, Razjouyan H, Etemadi A, Amjadi H, Merat S, Malekzadeh R. Ulcerative colitis and irritable bowel syndrome:

relationships with quality of life. *Eur J Gastroenterol Hepatol* 2008; 20: 46-50.

[74] Smrèn M, Axelsson J, Gillberg R, Abrahamsson H, Svedlund J, Björnsson ES. Quality of life in inflammatory bowel disease in remission: the impact of IBS-like symptoms and associated psychological factors. *Am J Gastroenterol* 2002; 97: 389-396.

[75] Minderhound IM, Oldenburg B, Wismeijer JA, Van Berge Henegouwen GP, Smout A. IBS-like symptoms in patients with inflammatory bowel disease in remission; relationship with quality of life and coping behavior. *Dig Dis Sci* 2004; 49: 469-474.

[76] Keohane J, O`Mahony C, O`Mahony L, O`Mahony S, Quilgley EM, Shanahan F. Irritable bowel syndrome-type symptoms in patients with inflammatory bowel disease: a real association or relation of occult inflammation. *Am J Gastroenterol* 2010; 105: 1789-1794.

[77] El-Salhy M, Danielsson Å, Stenling R, Grimelius L. Colonic endocrine cells in inflammatory bowel disease. *J Int Med* 1997; 242: 413-419.

[78] Böttcher G, Alumets J, Håkanson R, Sundler F. Co-existance of glicentin and peptide YY in colorectal L-cells in cat and man. An electron microscopic study. *Regul Pept* 1986; 13: 283-291.

[79] Böttcher G, Sjölund K, Ekblad E, Håkanson R, Schwarts TW, Sundler F. Co-existance of peptide YY and glicentin immunoreactivity in endocrine cells of the gut. *Regul Pept* 1984; 8: 261-266.

[80] Ali-Rachedi A, Varndell MI, Adrian TE, Gapp DA, van Noorden S, Bloom SR, Polak JM. Peptide YY (PYY) immunoreactivity is co-stored with glucagon-related immunoreactants in endocrine cells of the gut and pancreas. *Histochemistry* 1984; 80: 487-491.

[81] Nilsson O, Bilchik AJ, Goldenring JR, Ballantyne GH, Adrian TE, Modlin IM. Distribution and immunocytochemical colocalization of peptide YY and enteroglucagon in endocrine cells of the rabbit colon. *Endocrinology* 1991; 129: 139-148.

[82] Stoyanova II, Gulubova MV. Mast cells and inflammatory mediators in chronic ulcerative colitis. *Acta Histochem* 2002; 104: 185-192.

[83] Coates MD, Mahoney CR, Linden DR, Sampson JE, Chen J, Blaszyk H, Crowell MD, Sharkey KA, Greshon MD, Mawe GM, Moses PL. Molecular defects in mucosal serotonin content and decreased serotonin reuptake transporter in ulcerative colitis and irritable bowel syndrome. *Gastroenterology* 2004; 126: 1657-1664.

[84] Shi-Jun L, Yu-Qing L, Jian-Shao L, Hong-Juan W, Yong-Hong S, Yu-Bin T. VIP immunoreactive nerve and somatostatin and serotonin

containing cells in Crohn's disease. *World J Gastroenterol* 1999; 5: 541-543.

[85] Tari A, Teshima H, Sumii K, Haruma K, Ohgoshi H, Yoshihara M, Kajiyama G, Miyachi Y. Peptide YY abnormalities in patients with ulcerative colitis. *Jpn J Med* 1988; 27: 49-55.

[86] Qian B-F , El-Salhy M, Melgar S, Hammarström M-L. Danielsson Å. Neuroendocrine changes in colon of mice with a disrupted IL-2 gene. *Clin Exp Immunoø* 2000; 120: 424-433.

[87] Hirotani Y, Mikajiri K, Ikeda K, Myotoku M, Kurokawa N. Changes in the peptide YY levels in the intestinal tissue of rats with experimental colitis following oral administration of Mesalazine and prednisolon. Yakugaku Zasshi 2008; 128: 1347-1353.

[88] Surrenti C, Renzi MR, surreni E, Salvadori G. Colonic vasoactive intestinal polypeptides in ulcerative colitis. *J Physiol* 1993; 87: 307-311.

[89] Yukawa T, Oshitani N, Yamagami H, Watanabe K, Higuchi K, Arakawa T. Differntial expression of vasoactive intestinal receptor 1 expression in inflammatory bowel disease. *Int J Mol Med* 2007; 20: 161-167.

[90] Lee CM, Kumar RK, Lubowski DZ, Brucher E. Neuropeptides and nerve growth in inflammatory bowel diseases: a quantitative immunohistochemical study. *Dig Dis Sci* 2002; 47: 495-502.

[91] Cermon AM, Santini D, Cogliandro RF, De Giorgio R, Stanghellini V, Corinaldesi R, Barbara G. Mucosa immune activation in irritable bowel syndrome gender-dependence and association with digestive symptoms. *Am J Gastroenterol* 2009; 104: 392-400.

[92] Zucchelli M, Camilleri M, Andeasson AN, Bresso F, Dlugosz A, Halfvarson J, Törkvist L, Schmidt PT, Karling P, Ohlsson B, Duerr RH, Simren M, Lindberg G, Agreus L, Carlson P, Zinsmeister A, D`Amato M. Association of *TNFSF15* polymorphism with irritable bowel syndrome. *Gut* 2011; 60: 1671-1677.

Chapter VI

Treatment Options

Abstract

The options for the treatment of IBS are non-pharmacological and pharmacological.

The non-pharmacological approach comprises: information, reassurance, dietary guidance, regular exercise, probiotic intake, gut-directed hypnotherapy, cognitive therapy, acupuncture and herbal therapy. Pharmacological treatment depends on the symptoms and mainly includes anti-diarrhoeal drugs, laxatives, antispasmodic drugs, antidepressants, anti-anxiety drugs and antibiotics. General practitioners and gastroenterologists use non-pharmacological approaches and pharmacological drugs to the same extent. Patient confidence is higher with the non-pharmacological approach than with medication, and the non-pharmacological approach is more effective than medication. Of the non-pharmacological approaches, information, reassurance, dietary guidance, regular exercise, probiotic intake and gut-directed hypnotherapy have been proven to be effective in the management of IBS and to improve symptoms and quality of life. Anti-diarrhoeal drugs, laxatives and antidepressant drugs also proved to be effective in the management of IBS.

Introduction

The treatment options for IBS include non-pharmacological and pharmacological options [1]. The non-pharmacological approach comprises:

information, reassurance, dietary guidance, regular exercise, probiotic intake, hypnotherapy and cognitive therapy, amongst others [1-4]. Pharmacological treatment mainly includes laxatives, anti-diarrhoeal drugs, antispasmodic drugs, antidepressants and anti-anxiety drugs [1-4]. The use of non-pharmacological treatments and pharmacological drugs in primary health care and by gastroenterologists is almost the same (Figures 27 and 28) [1]. Patient confidence is higher for the non-pharmacological approach than medication, and the non-pharmacological approach is also more effective than medication [1].

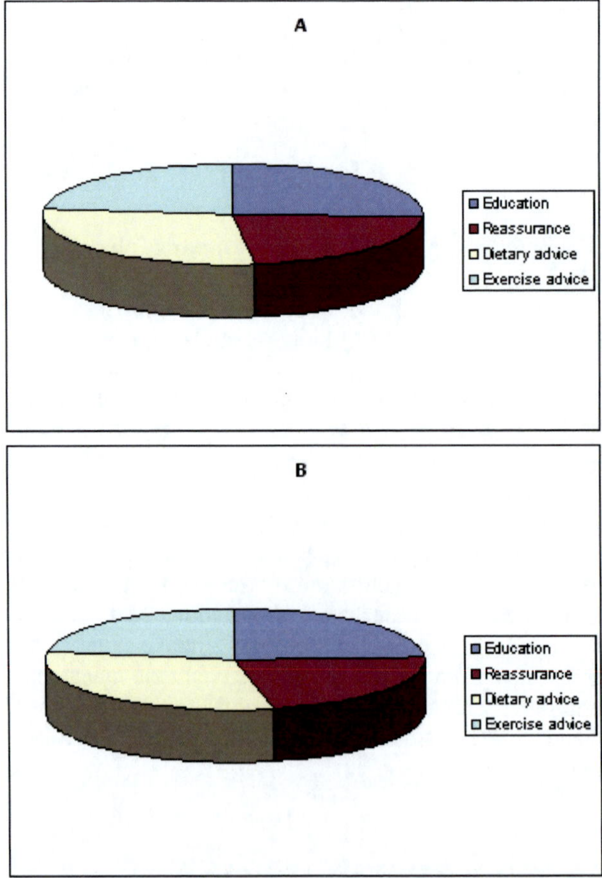

Figure 27. No difference was found between GPs (A) and Specialists (B) regarding the non-pharmacological approach for managing IBS patients.

6.1. Non-Pharmacological Approaches

6.1.1. Information and Reassurance

In order to investigate what patients with IBS know about IBS and what they would like to know, a survey was conducted on 1242 IBS patients [5]. This survey showed that 52% believed that IBS is caused by a lack of digestive enzymes, 42.8% believed that IBS is a form of colitis, 47.9% believed it will worsen with age and 43% believed it can develop into colitis, 37.7% malnutrition and 21.4% cancer [5]. The same patients were interested in learning about which foods to avoid (63.3%), the causes of IBS (62%), coping strategies (59.4%) and medications (55.2%); they were also interested in finding out whether or not they would have to live with IBS for life (51.6%) and in reading research studies (48.6%) [5]. The most desired qualities in health-care providers according to the IBS patients were the ability to provide comprehensive information (96%), to refer to a source for additional information (95.8%), to answer questions (95.9%), to listen (94.4%), to provide information about IBS studies and medications (94%) and to provide support (88.6%) and hope (82.1%) [6]. However, the previous experiences of IBS patients with their health-care providers were quite different from their expectations [6]. Not surprisingly, IBS patients reporting experiencing dissatisfaction and negative attitudes in their contact with health-care providers (see Chapter 1). Patient dissatisfaction stemmed from the actual information provided and how this was communicated [7]. A rather interesting finding was that the majority of the IBS patients stated that they prefer to get information from a doctor in person [5, 8, 9]. In a survey of 1242 IBS patients, it was found that the most desired source of information was "my doctor" (68%), followed by the internet (62%) and information leaflets (45%) [9].

An effective physician-patient relationship that provides both reassurance and a thorough explanation of the IBS disorder has been found to reduce the use of health-care resources and the fear of cancer [10-13]. A 15-minute thorough oral explanation of the diagnosis and underlying mechanisms of IBS and a complete physical examination by a gastroenterologist during the first consultation was found to reduce self-perceptions of impairment in daily functioning [14]. Furthermore, a structured 3-hour IBS educational class for patients with IBS was reported to improve symptoms and some health-promoting behaviours [15]. In an ambitious 12-hour structured IBS educational programme, including a 2-hour informative session with a gastroenterologist, was found to improve both symptoms and quality of life [16, 17].

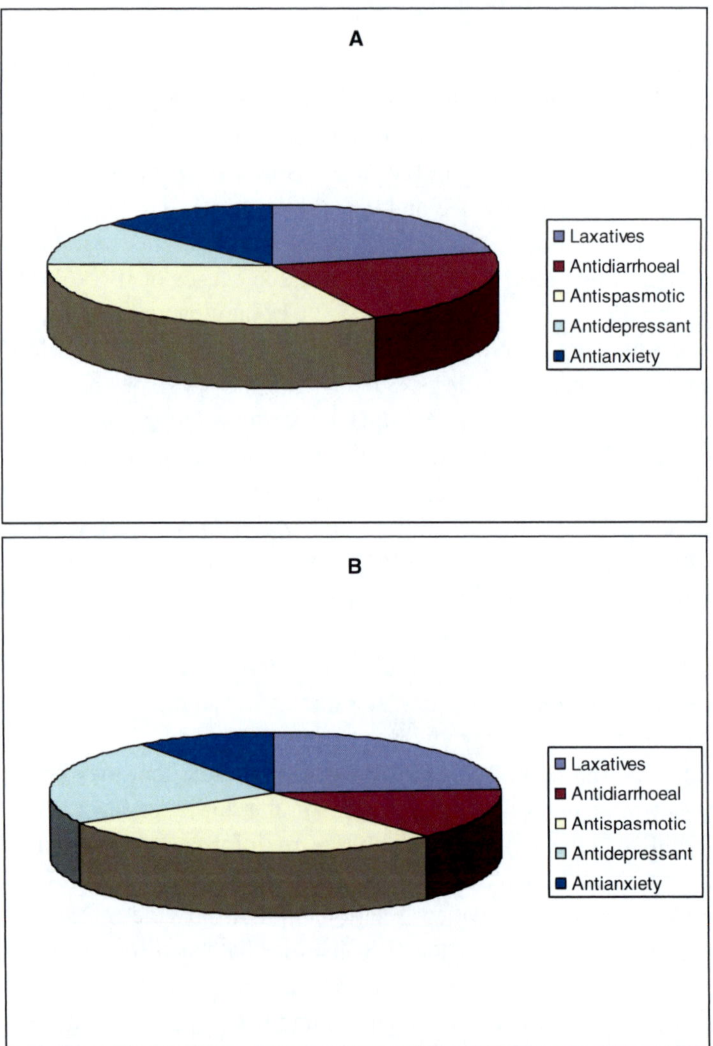

Figure 28. The GPs (A) prescribed the same proportions of pharmacological treatment to the IBS patients as the specialists (B).

It is clear from what is mentioned above that information and education are both requested by IBS patients and have been proven to be beneficial; however, several aspects should be considered. In which way and by whom should information and reassurance be given to IBS patients? Should it be done by the patient's doctor during a consultation or in a group by a team of health-care professionals including a doctor (IBS school)? What information and other measures should be taken to reassure IBS patients?

We believe that information and reassurance should be provided by the patient's doctor simply because this is what the patients prefer. Moreover, this is important in establishing patient-doctor relationships. Consequently, these patients need longer consultations than normal. This is likely to prove a problem with fixed-timed appointments. Dedicated, longer time slots may be an appropriate way to manage the disorder rather than repeated brief consultations. Actually, this approach would not be very time-consuming than when doctors offer group sessions [16,17], as 2 hours of a gastroenterologist's time are used to inform a group of 5-7 patients [16,17]. One of the arguments in favour of providing information to a small group of patients has been that patient education in a group setting offers an opportunity to share experiences with others in the same situation, which can contribute to improvements in coping strategies [17]. The authors further explained that, according to the self-efficacy theory, one of the best ways of enhancing self-efficacy and changes in behaviour is to see someone else with the same problem making such changes (modelling) [17]. As a matter of fact, modelling, according to the self-efficacy theory, is a process of comparing oneself with someone else. When people see someone succeeding at something, their self-efficacy is more likely to increase, whereas when they see people failing their self-efficacy is more likely to decrease. This process is more effective when a person sees him- or herself as being similar to his or her own model. Regarding this matter, the IBS patients who attended the IBS School apparently failed to cope with IBS, according to the modelling, seeing failed people is more likely to decrease self-efficacy. In one IBS school where a huge amount of resources were used (six 2-h sessions with a nurse, a gastroenterologist, a physiotherapist and a psychologist), the outcome was rather poor. Although improvements were shown in the symptoms up to 6 months, there were no further improvements after 1 year and the overall quality of life score did not improve at all, except temporarily in a few dimensions [17].

Optimal consultation techniques designed to elicit a therapeutic alliance between patients and physicians, which should be applied in all physician consultations, are especially important in consultations with IBS patients. The patients should be allowed to tell their story in their own words in order to feel that the doctor has understood their concerns. This becomes even more important when previous consultations may have been unsatisfactory in this respect. Furthermore, the first consultation should include the provision of detailed information regarding IBS, a thorough physical examination and some blood tests to exclude infection/inflammation, anaemia, diabetes, or thyroidal, liver or kidney diseases.

The information provided to the patients should include the following:

- Irritable bowel syndrome is a common disorder in the population and is more common in women than in men, and there is some evidence to show that it could be hereditary. Irritable bowel syndrome is recognized as an illness.
- Irritable bowel syndrome is not known to be associated with the development of serious disease or with excess mortality.
- Irritable bowel syndrome is a chronic disorder and the intensity of symptoms fluctuate, i.e., there will be good days and bad days.
- A clear knowledgeable explanation of the pathophysiology and the pathogenesis of IBS.
- The possible co-existence of other gastrointestinal and extra-gastrointestinal symptoms in patients with IBS.
- A thorough explanation regarding the fact that a physical examination, blood tests, gastroscopy and colonoscopy can exclude other diseases that the patients fear (see Chapter 3). In patients who have already undergone gastroscopy and colonoscopy, an explanation should be offered as to what these tests have excluded.
- An explanation of the treatment options and the fact that a non-pharmacological approach could be sufficient and could be combined with pharmacological treatment on bad days. It should be clearly stated that there is no miracle cure.
- Intensive research is being carried out on IBS worldwide and our understanding of this disorder increases every day, which will hopefully offer new treatment possibilities. In other words, there will be light at the end of the tunnel.

An educational booklet containing the same information should be freely available at the end of the consultation, along with the opportunity for patients to discuss their concerns again once they have read this material.

Another aspect to consider is the follow-up of these patients. The majority of IBS patients would like to be followed up; this represents an important factor regarding the reassurance of patients, whereby they feel that on bad days they can obtain the support they need. In our clinic we offered a short consultation once a year; however, considering the size of this group of patients and the amount of resources declined, we were not able to provide this and instead informed them that they could phone and ask for an appointment whenever they needed it, without being refereed by a GP. In fact, a few patients asked for a new appointment as a result of drastic change in their life combined with severe abdominal symptoms.

The short consultation given to these few patients prevented hospitalization, numerous investigations and possibly unnecessary operations.

6.1.2. Dietary Guidance and Regular Exercise

Diet seems to play an important role in the manifestation of IBS symptoms. The mechanisms thought to lie behind this were discussed earlier (see Chapter 4). A restricted intake of FODMAPs has been shown to reduce symptoms of IBS [18,19]. An increased consumption of dietary fibre is thought to accelerate oro-anal transit time and decrease intracolonic pressure, therefore playing a role in the management of IBS symptoms, particularly regarding constipation [20]. However, more recent studies have yielded controversial results [21-23].

In these trials [21-23], dietary fibre was considered as a whole entity. In studies that distinguished between insoluble and soluble fibre, soluble fibre tended to improve symptoms whereas insoluble fibre worsened them [24]. Moreover, a recent, randomized, double-blind, placebo-controlled trial of soluble fibres showed a significant reduction in the intensity of abdominal pain, constipation and diarrhoea, as well as an improvement in the performance of daily activities [25]. A lower intake of FODMAPs should be recommended to IBS patients, as well as increasing their intake of foods rich in water soluble fibres (Table 5).

In the clinic, tolerance to FODMAPs and insoluble fibres varies between different patients with IBS. This wide variation could be due to differences in intestinal flora between patients.

Furthermore, consuming food supplemented with probiotics increases a patient's tolerance to FODMAPs and insoluble fibres. In addition to general dietary advice, individual dietary guidance is also required.

Table 5. General food advice to IBS patients

Food allowed	Food advised to avoid
Spelt and spelt products	Flour and four products
Meat	Onion
Fish	Garlic
Chicken	Paprika
Fat and oils	Cabbage and rutabaga
Rice	Carbonated beverages (soda)
Potatoes	Light products (food containing
Carrot	artificial sweeteners)
Apple and pear (peeled)	Beans
Citrus	Peas
Banana	Avocado
Raspberry blueberry and strawberry	Artichokes
Honeydew melon	Broccoli, cabbage
Kiwifruit and passion fruit	watermelon
Tomato	
Milk	
Coffee, tea	
Chocolate	
Alcohol	
Probiotic supplemented	

The IBS patients received two 1-hour sessions of individual dietary guidance recommending that they increase their daily intake of dairy products and food items supplemented with probiotics (Figure 25) [26]. They subsequently increased their intake of beta-carotene, retinol equivalents, riboflavin, calcium, magnesium and phosphorus (Figure 26) [26]. Furthermore, they reported a better quality of life and fewer symptoms (Figures 27 and 28) [26].

Regular exercise has been found to reduce symptoms and improve the quality of life in patients with IBS, [27-30]. Based on clinical experience and circumstantial evidence physicians recommended exercise for IBS patients. Physical activity effects on IBS patients have previously been attributed to promoting overall well being. However, Physical activity has been found to increase gastrointestinal transit [31, 32]. Furthermore, in high-endurance athletes there are a high prevalence of lower gastrointestinal symptoms, such as bloating, cramps and diarrhoea [33]. The increased gastrointestinal motility has been attributed to vagus stimulation and/or decreased blood flow to the gut, which leads to increase in important gastrointestinal hormones [32, 33].

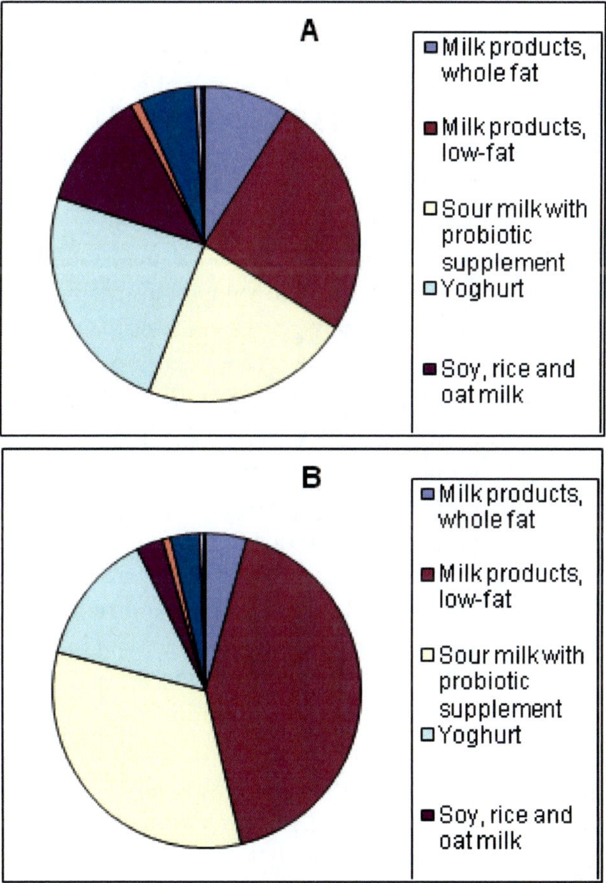

Figure 29. The daily intake of dairy products of IBS patients (A) and IBS patients 2 years after receiving 2 hours of individual dietary guidance (B).Data from [26].

6.1.3. Probiotics

Probiotics are live microorganisms that when administered in adequate amounts confer health benefits to the host [34]. The most commonly used probiotics include bacteria or yeasts from the genera *Lactobacillus*, *Bidifobacteria* and *Saccharomyces* [35]. Commercially available probiotics contain either single strains or a mixture of strains and are available in capsules, powders, yoghurts and fermented milks. Probiotics must be well tolerated for human consumption, they must survive transit through the gastrointestinal tract and they must have some physiological impact. Some of the beneficial effects attributed to probiotics are enhancement of the host's anti-inflammatory and immune response and the stimulation of anti-inflammatory cytokines, improving the epithelial cell barrier, inhibiting bacterial translocation and growth, inhibiting the adhesion of viruses and inactivating bile acids [36, 37]. In animal models, probiotics have been found to reduce hypermotility and visceral hypersensitivity [36].

Controlled clinical trials of a single probiotic preparation [38-47] and a probiotic mixture [48-53] showed that IBS symptoms are improved depending on the preparation used, and that some products appear to be more effective than others [35-37,54]. The bacteria that have been proven to be effective in this aspect are *Bifidobacterium infantis* 35624, *Bifidobacterium lactis* DN-173-010, *L. plantrum*, L. GG, *L. acidophilus* and *S. faecium* [35-37, 55]. The mechanism that seems to lay behind this improvement is the ability of these bacteria to reduce the number of sulphite-reducing *Clostridia* spp., which is known to produce gas upon the fermentation of nutrients. This could contribute to improvements in flatulence, bloating and abdominal distension in IBS patients [37]. Furthermore, the anti-inflammatory and immune-modulating responses shown might be important factors [36,37] regarding the notion that low-grade inflammation plays a role in the aetiology of IBS [see Chapter 4].

Although probiotics have beneficial effects in some patients with IBS, they are not potent enough to be used alone, especially in patients with severe symptoms [36]. It is noteworthy that, in clinical practice, a relapse of IBS symptoms was observed in some patients as soon as they stopped taking the probiotics [56]. This clinical observation was supported by the fact that, 1 week after stopping the probiotic, *Lactobacillus acidophilus* vanished from the faeces [56]; thus, probiotics should be taken continuously.

Prebiotics are defined as non-digestible, fermentable food components that result in the selective stimulation and/or activity of one or a limited number of microbial genera/species in the gut microbiota that confer health benefits to the host [57]. Prebiotics are only fermented by a limited number of genera/species, which subsequently increase in number via natural selection from the carbon and energy afforded by prebiotics. The benefits of the use of prebiotics in IBS are not yet clear, but they probably represent a potential tool for the management of IBS [35, 37].

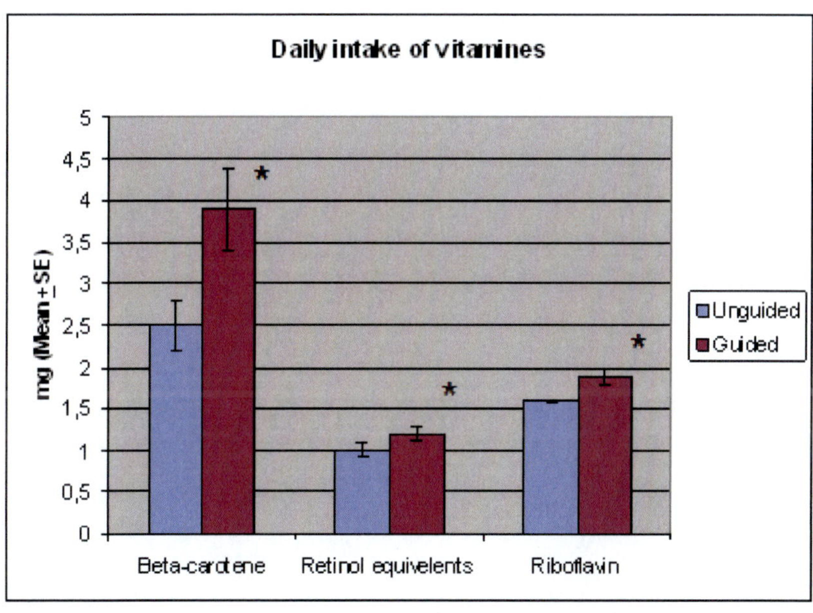

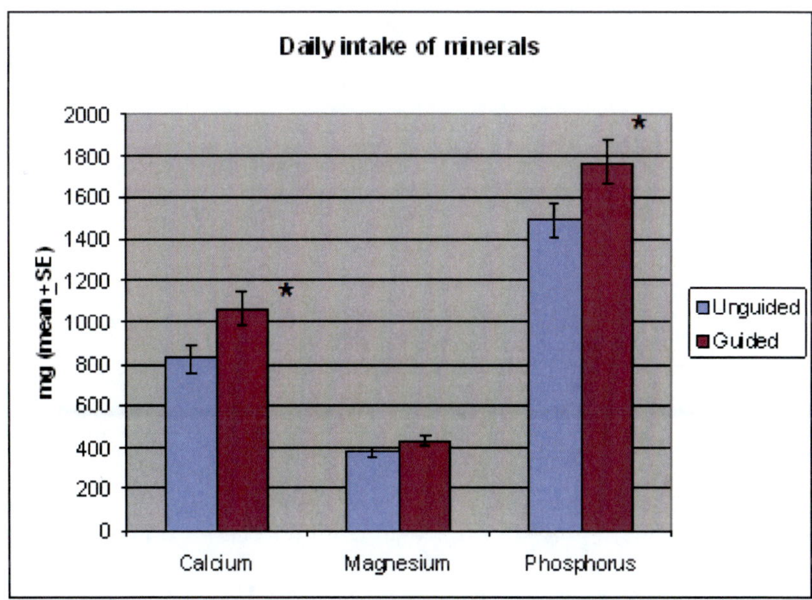

Figure 30. After 2 years, the IBS patients who received 2 hours of individual dietary guidance had increased their daily intake of vitamins and minerals more than the IBS patients who did not receive any dietary guidance. Data from [26].

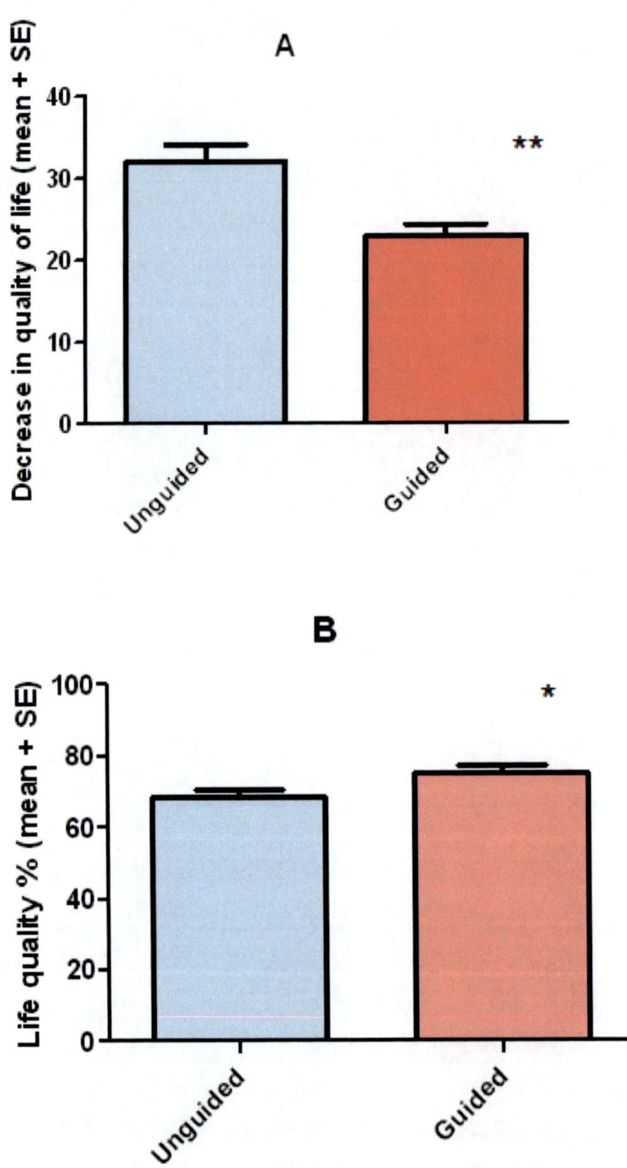

*=P<0.05; **=P<0.01. Data from 26.

Figure 31. After 2 years, the IBS patients who received 2 hours of individual dietary guidance had a higher quality of life according to the Short-Form Nepean Dyspepsia Index (SF-NDI) (A) and Irritable Bowel Syndrome Quality Of Life (IBS-QOL) (B) than the IBS patients who did not receive any dietary guidance.

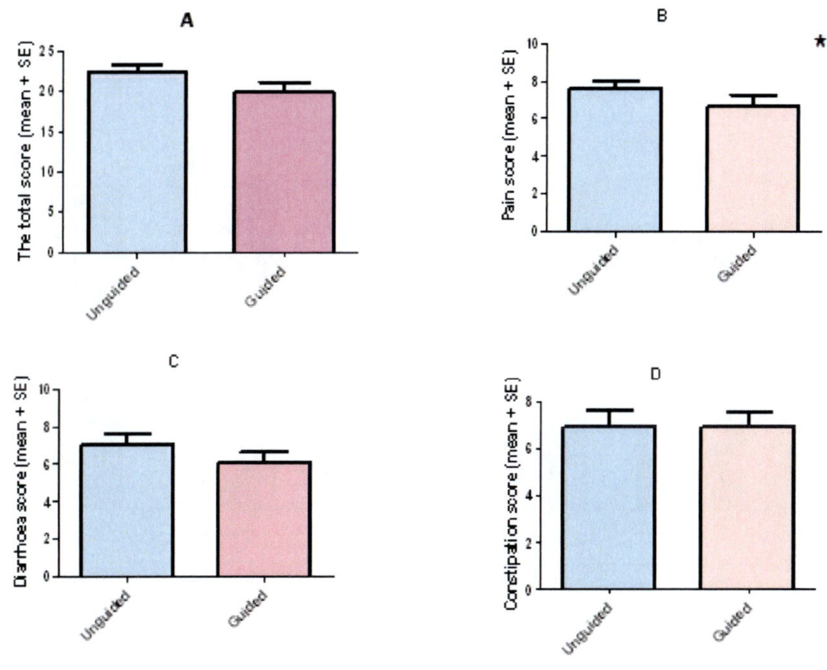

*=P<0.05. Data from 26.

Figure 32. After 2 years, the IBS patients who received 2 hours of individual dietary guidance showed greater improvements in their IBS symptoms according to the Birmingham IBS symptom questionnaire than the IBS patients who did not receive any dietary guidance.

6.1.4. Combined Programme

As mentioned above, the provision of reassurance and information, dietary management, probiotic intake and regular exercise have been found to reduce symptoms and improve quality of life in IBS patients. A health programme combining these elements was followed by 143 IBS patients, who were followed up over 2 years [55]. It was found that combining reassurance and information, dietary management, probiotic intake and regular exercise seemed to have an additive effect, and the patients who followed this programme reported an improved quality of life (Figure 29) and reduced symptoms (Figure 30) throughout the follow-up period [55]. These findings are in favour of the additive effect of combining several non-pharmacological approaches in a short health programme. Data from 55.

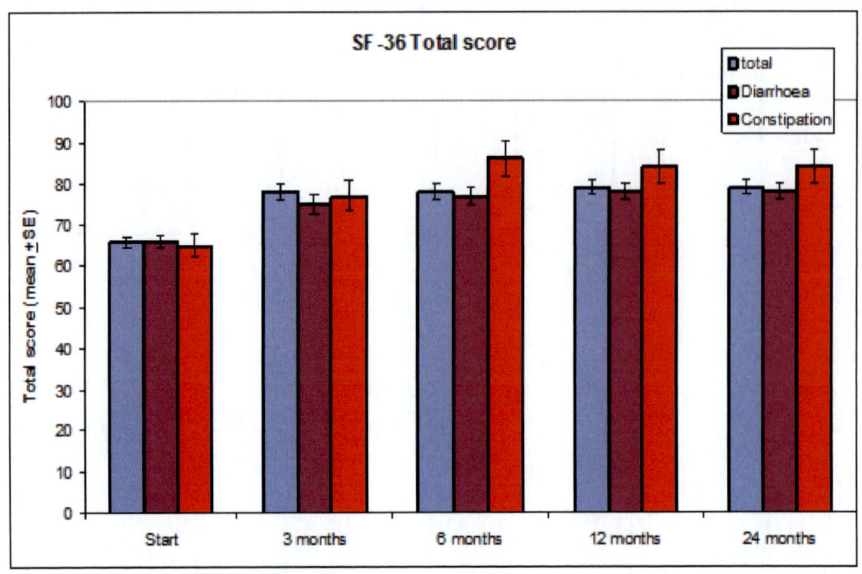

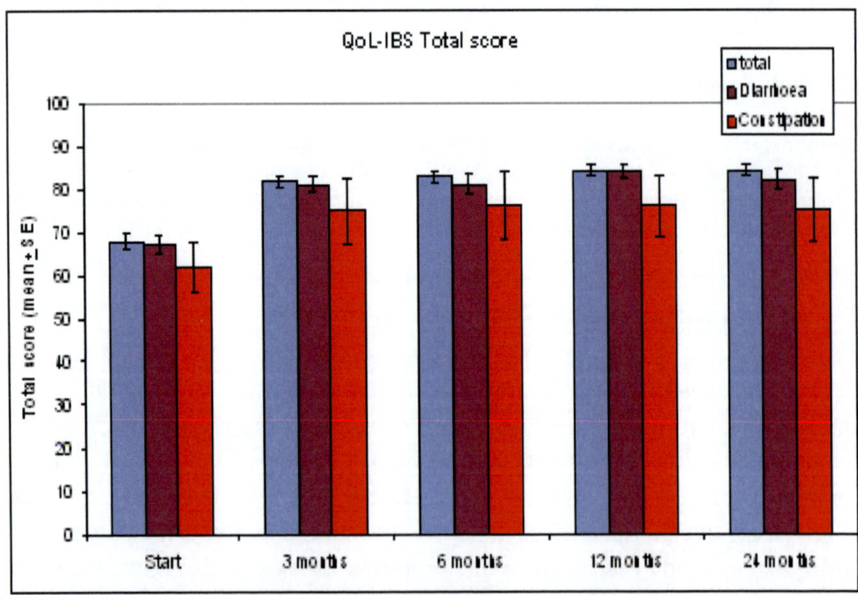

Figure 33. Quality of life in IBS patients who underwent a health programme comprising reassurance and information, dietary management, probiotic intake and regular exercise. Data from 55.

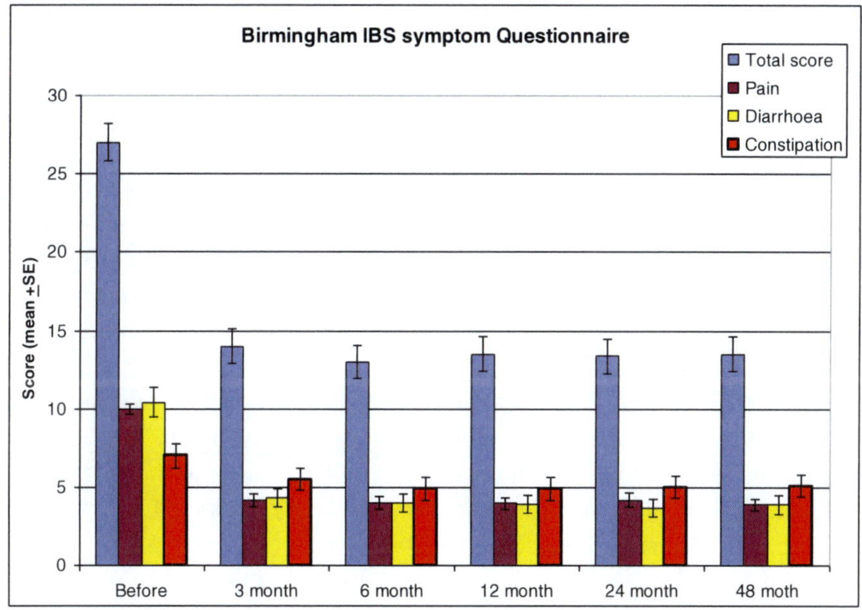

Figure 34. Symptom reduction in IBS patients who underwent a health programme comprising reassurance and information, diet management, probiotic intake and regular exercise.

6.1.5. Psychological Treatment

There is still some uncertainty regarding the role of psychological therapy in managing IBS [4]. This is due to significant challenges in terms of study design, patient selection and the interpretation of results.

6.1.5.1. Gut-Directed Hypnotherapy

Gut-directed hypnotherapy is based on the use of hypnotic induction, using progressive relaxation and other techniques, followed by imagery directed towards the control and normalization of gut functions [58-61]. Therapy also aims to teach autohypnosis in order to enable patients to manage their own symptoms without ongoing reliance on health-care. Occasional refresher sessions, however, may be required [61]. Gut-directed hypnotherapy is a time-intensive intervention, requiring a total of about 6 to 12 sessions, each between 30 and 60 min long, over a period of several months [61]. The dropout rates in patients with refractory IBS are relatively high [61]. A home hypnosis programme (delivered on five compact disks) could be useful, but the response rate to this type of therapy is generally not as high as that of therapist-led treatment [62].

Gut-directed hypnotherapy has been shown to be effective not only in improving IBS symptoms but also in improving many of the features of the condition, including quality of life and psychological status [59,61,63,64]. Moreover, the beneficial effects appear to be sustained over time, with patients reporting continued relief from symptoms for at least five years [63]. It is noteworthy that these results were mostly based on patients in secondary care and that the majority were refractory (patients with severe symptoms and long duration of IBS) cases of IBS and were highly selected slightly older and motivated IBS patients. The results of the studies mentioned here cannot be generalized to IBS patients as a whole. This type of treatment is extremely operator dependent and therefore subject to variations in the quality of provision [61,65]. This form of treatment should be restricted to specialist centres caring for more severe forms of IBS [61].

Gut-directed hypnotherapy normalizes visceral sensation [66], reduces colonic phasic contractions [67] and reverses the negative thoughts that patients often have regarding their condition [68]. It has been proposed that the action of hypnotherapy is probably due to the activation of certain areas of the brain, especially the anterior cingulated, which is supported by the finding that the hypnotic reduction of somatic pain is associated with a reduction in the activation of this brain region [68].

6.1.5.2. Cognitive Behaviour, Psychodynamic Interpersonal Therapies and Relaxation Training

Cognitive behavioural therapy is based on two central underlying assumptions: 1. symptoms are acquired (learned) and reflect specific skills deficits in cognitive and behavioural functioning, and 2. teaching and rehearsing skills for modifying maladaptive behaviours and thinking patterns can remediate these deficits, which, in turn, relieve symptoms. The evidence for the efficacy of cognitive behavioural therapy remains controversial [69-74]. Whereas satisfaction and global well being are improved, little effect has been found on abdominal pain or IBS-specific quality of life. Some authors have claimed that cognitive behavioural therapy has a direct effect on global IBS symptom improvement independent of its effect on distress and that these improvements are not moderated by variables reflecting the mental well being of IBS patients [73]. Others claim that this improvement is due to indirect pathways that operate via mood, most clearly anxiety but also, to a lesser extent, depression [74]. The common belief, however, is that cognitive behavioural therapy may help patients cope with their symptoms without necessarily abolishing them [4].

Psychodynamic interpersonal therapy attempts to help the patient understand how their emotional state is related to stress and the link between emotions and bowel symptoms. This is brought about by providing the patient with insights into why symptoms develop in the context of difficulties or changes in key relationships [75]. This treatment could lead to significant life changes and to improvements in the emotional state, IBS symptoms and quality of life [75-78].

It is unclear how much of the benefit of relaxation training is due to increased attention from the therapist [79-81]. Relaxation training includes yoga meditation, biofeedback and progressive muscle relaxation [82, 83]. This approach can be useful in patients for whom stress is an important factor in triggering IBS symptoms.

6.2. Pharmacological Approaches

6.2.1. Symptomatic Treatment

Pharmacological treatments for the relief of IBS symptoms have been presented in detail in recent comprehensive reviews [4, 84-87]. Drug treatment is chosen based on the main symptoms that trouble patients; thus, pharmacological drugs against abdominal pain and/or bloating, diarrhoea and constipation are most commonly used (Table 6).

Diarrhoea in IBS patients can be treated with loperamide or diphenoxylate. Loperamide is an opiate μ-agonist that does not cross the blood-brain barrier. It is widely used in clinical practice because it is effective for urgent loose stools and it is safe, well tolerated and inexpensive [88]. Loperamide stimulates absorption, inhibits secretion and slows intestinal transit. However, it is not effective on abdominal pain [89].

Several tricyclic antidepressants are used to treat IBS patients, especially those with diarrhoea as the predominant symptom. These have anticholinergic and non-selective serotonin reuptake inhibitor effects. These drugs may alter pain perception [90, 91] independent of their antidepressant or anxiety effects [92]. However, even treatment with low doses of these drugs can cause side effects such as a dry mouth, constipation, fatigue and drowsiness in over one third of patients. Selective serotonin reuptake inhibitors inhibit the reuptake of serotonin by blocking the serotonin transporter protein at presynaptic nerve endings and increasing synaptic exposure to a high concentration of serotonin [93]. A standard dose of selective serotonin reuptake inhibitors has been shown to lead to a significant improvement in health-related quality of life in patients with chronic or treatment-resistant IBS [94]. These drugs confer global benefits without significant changes in bowel symptoms or pain [94-97]. These drugs are better tolerated by patients than tricyclic antidepressants.

Table. 6. Pharmacological options for the treatment of IBS patients

Drug class	Generic name	The target symptom	Dose
Opiate μ-agonist	Loperamide	Diarrhoea	2 mg with each loose stool, to maximum 16 mg/d
Tricyclic antidepressants	Desipramide	Diarrhoea, abdominal distension and pain	10-150 mg at night
	Amitriptyline		10-150 mg at night
	Nortriptyline		10-150 mg at night
Selective serotonin reuptake inhibitors	Paroxetine	Global benefit without benefit to bowel symptoms	20-50 mg daily
	Fluoxetine		10-40 mg daily
Antibiotics	Rifaximin	Global improvement of symptoms and improvement in bloating and distension	400-550 mg three times daily in 7-10 days
	Neomycin		1 g daily in 10 days
	Metronidazol		400 mg twice daily in 15 days
Bulking agents	Psyllium	Improve straining and hard stools	2.5-30 g daily in divided doses
	Ispaghula		3.5 g one to three times daily
Osmotic laxative	Polyethylene glycol		17 g in 237 ml solution daily
Emollient laxative	Mineral oil		5-10 cm^3 daily
Antispasmodics	Hysocamine sulfate	Limited proven efficacy	0.125 mg up to four times daily
	Dicyclomine		10-20 mg twice to four times daily

The rationale for using antibiotics in the treatment of IBS is based on the assumption that IBS symptoms could be caused by small intestinal bacterial overgrowth and the presence of inflammatory mediators and/or inflammatory cells in the mucosa of some IBS patients [98]. Clinical trials with antibiotics have shown global relief of IBS symptoms and bloating [98-104].

Several treatment options are available for the symptomatic relief of constipation in IBS patients [4,91-104]. Soluble fibres and bulking agents are most frequently used as the first-line treatment; conventional bulking agents include psyllium, methylcellulose and calcium polycarbophil. Bulking agents containing insoluble fibres have often the adverse effects of bloating and flatulence. Psyllium and ispaghula (a derivative of psyllium) have been proven to be effective and free from the side effects of other bulking agents [105-108]. Osmotic laxatives such as polyethylene glycol and lactulose are used for constipation in IBS, although lactulose is associated with bloating and abdominal pain and is not suitable for chronic use. Stimulant laxatives as bisacodyl and senna are effective but are associated with abdominal cramping, electrolyte depletion and diarrhoea [109], and consequently should not be used for long periods.

The rationale behind the use of an antispasmodic agent is to attenuate the heightened baseline and postprandial contractility observed in IBS patients; however, the efficacy of these agents in the treatment of IBS is limited [110-113].

In randomised, double blind, placebo controlled studies, administration of 3 mg melatonin at bedtime attenuated abdominal pain and reduced rectal pain sensitivity. This treatment have no effect on sleep disturbances or psychological stress suggesting that the beneficial effects of melatonin are independent of its action on sleep disturbances or psychological profiles [114, 115].

6.2.2. The Use of Gut Neuroendocrine Peptides/Amines in the Treatment of IBS

The neuroendocrine peptides/amines of the gut have the potential to be used in the treatment of IBS; this could be considered as the correction of a pre-existing abnormality through the use of the pharmacological actions of these substances. The problem with using the neuroendocrine peptides/amines of the gut as drugs is that, by their very nature, they have broad physiological/pharmacological effects: they can often bind to and activate several receptors with independent actions. Thus, in order to be able to target these bioactive substances, receptor-specific agonists or antagonists should be developed. Both serotonin agonists and antagonists have been proven to be useful in clinical practice. There are seven different families of 5-HT (serotonin) receptors and 21 different subtypes. Most of these receptors occur in the central nervous system. Only the 5-HT receptors 5-HT1, 5-HT3 and 5-HT4 are widely expressed in the gut [116-120].

The 5-HT1 receptors are expressed by a subset of inhibitory motor neurones of the myenteric plexus of the stomach [120,121]. Sumatriptan is a gastric 5-HT1p receptor agonist which relaxes the stomach and delays gastric emptying of solids and liquids [122-125]. Buspirone and R137696 are 5-HT1 receptor agonists with similar effects as sumatriptan [126-128]. These agonists have been found to improve the symptoms of early satiety in dyspeptic patients with impaired accommodation [128-130]. However, this 5-HT receptor does not seem to be clinically relevant as a target for the treatment of IBS patients.

Ondansetron, granisetron, aldosterone, and cilansetron are 5-HT3 receptor antagonists [130]. These antagonists have been found to decrease small intestinal secretion, small and large intestinal motility and nausea, as well as reducing colonic hypersensitivity [130-137]. Aldosterone was approved for the treatment of IBS-diarrhoea in female patients [138-142], but it was later withdrawn from the market because of side effects [143]. Other 5-HT3 receptor antagonists, especially cilansetron, have been investigated or are still under development for the treatment of IBS-diarrhoea patients [144-145]. In contrast, 5-HT3 receptor agonists have no therapeutic value because of their role in signalling nociceptive information from the bowel to the central nervous system, such as nausea [130].

The 5HT4 receptors are located on afferent neurones in the myenteric plexus, smooth muscles and enterochromaffin cells [146,147]. These receptors mediate the release of the colonic neurotransmitters acetylcholine, substance P, vasoactive intestinal polypeptide [VIP] and calcitonin-gene-related peptide, which stimulate the peristaltic reflex [148]. Furthermore, 5HT4 receptor activation induces small bowel and colonic fluid secretion [149-151]. Tegaserod, prucalopride, renzapride and cisapride are 5HT4 receptor agonists [130]. Tegasrode has been shown to promote small intestinal transit time and to enhance proximal colonic emptying in IBS-constipation patients [152]. In healthy humans, tegaserod stimulates intestinal secretion and promotes the evacuation of jejunely perfused gas [153-155]. Tegaserod has been used to treat IBS-constipation, but it was withdrawn from the market because of its side effects [154]. Prucalopride has been also been reported to decrease colonic transit time [155].

Ingested nutrients and their digestion products initiate local responses including the release of neuroendocrine peptides/amines in the gut [see Table 4]. The protein, fat and carbohydrate contents of ingested food influence the amount and type of gut hormone released. These hormones regulate and control gastrointestinal motility and sensation. Thus, pre-existed abnormalities in the neuroendocrine system of the gut could be compensated for through dietary manipulation, one could compensate pre-existed abnormalities in the neuroendocrine system of the gut. This approach appears to be successful [156-159].

6.3. Other Treatment Options

6.3.1. Acupuncture

Acupuncture is an ancient traditional Chinese medical practice [160] based on the theory that energy or the life force "qi" runs through the body in channels, or "meridians". Qi is essential for health and any disruption of its flow causes symptoms and disease.

This disruption is believed to be corrected by acupuncture at identifiable anatomical locations called "acupoints". The effect of acupuncture on IBS is believed to be caused by altering visceral sensation and motility by stimulating the somatic nervous system and vagus nerve [161-163].

Acupuncture intervention in a randomized controlled pilot study showed significant improvements in IBS symptoms [164]. A review of randomized trials using acupuncture for IBS found inconclusive evidence of the efficacy of this type of intervention [165]. In another two large, randomized controlled studies, no difference was found in the global outcome measurements between patients who received real or sham acupuncture [166,167].

However, improvements were found in IBS symptoms and quality of life in patients who received real and sham acupuncture compared to baseline values and IBS patients on the waiting list [166,167]. These findings suggest that the observed effect of acupuncture may have been due to the placebo effect.

6.3.2. Herbal Therapy

In traditional Chinese medical theory IBS is a syndrome of stagnated liver energy and a dysfunction of the spleen [168]. Thus, Chinese herbal treatments for IBS were developed to relieve suppressed liver functioning and to replenish the energy of the spleen [168,169]. There are several Chinese herbal formulations for IBS, such as Tong Yao Fang (the essential formula for abdominal pain and diarrhoea), which contains up to 20 herbal ingredients, and the Tibetan herbal formulation Padma Lax. Studies on the beneficial effects of herbal treatments have shown conflicting results [170-173] and the efficacy of this type of treatment remains controversial.

Steam distillation oil extracts from the peppermint plant (*Mentha piperita*, Lamiaceae) are among the oldest remedies for the treatment of gastrointestinal problems. These extracts are believed to improve IBS symptoms by exerting a spasmolytic effect on the smooth muscles of the digestive tract [174,175]. Most trials support the effectiveness of peppermint oil in improving IBS symptoms [176-180]; however, further studies are needed to elucidate the beneficial effects of such a treatment.

References

[1]   Whitehead WE, Levy RL, Von Korff M, Feld AD, Palsson OS, Turner M, Drossman DA. The usual medical care for irritable bowel syndrome. *Aliment Pharmacol Ther* 2004, 20: 1305-1315.

[2]   Yoon SL, Grundmann O, Koepp L, Farrell L. Mangement of irritable bowel syndrome (IBS) in adults: conventional and complementary /alternative approaches. *Altern Med Rev* 2011; 16: 134-151.

[3]   Spiller RC. Treatment of irritable bowel syndrome. *Current Treatment Options in Gastroenterology* 2003; 6: 329-337.

[4]   Spiller R, Aziz Q, Creed F, Emmanuel A, Houghton L, Hungin P, Jones R, Kumor D, Rubin G, Trudgill N, Whorwell P. Guidelines on the irritable bowel syndrome: mechanisms and practical management. *Gut* 2007; 56: 1770-1798.

[5]   Halpert A, Dalton CB, Palsson O, Morris C, HU Y, Bangiwala S, Hankins J, Norton N, Drossman D. What patients know about irritable bowel syndrome (IBS) and what they would like to know. National survey on patients educational needs in IBS and development and

validation of the patient educational needs questionnaire (PEQ). *Am J Gastroenterol* 2007; 102: 1972-1982.

[6] Halpert A, Dalton CB, Palsson O, Morris C, HU Y, Bangiwala S, Hankins J, Norton N, Drossman D. Irritable bowel syndrome.Patients' ideal expectations and recent experiences with healthcare providers. a national survey. *Dig Dis Sci* 2010; 55: 375-383.

[7] Dhaliwal SK, Hunt RH. Doctor-patient interaction for irritable bowel syndrome in primary care: a systematic perspective. *Eur J Gastroenterol Hepatol* 2004; 16: 116-166.

[8] Halpert A, Thomas AC, HU Y, Morris CB, Bangiwala SI, Drossman DA. A survey on patients educational needs in irritable bowel syndrome and attitudes toward participation in clinical research. *J Clin Gastroenterol* 2006; 40: 37-43.

[9] Halpert A, Dalton CB, Palsson O, Morris C, HU Y, Bangiwala S, Hankins J, Norton N, Drossman DA. Patient educational media preference for information about irritable bowel syndrome (IBS). *Dig Dis Sci* 2008; 53: 184-190.

[10] Drossman DA, Patrick DL, Whitehead WE,Toner BB, Diamant NE, Hu Y, Jia H, Bangdiwala SI. Further validation of the IBS-QOL: a disease-specific quality-of-life questionnaire. *Am J Gastroenterol* 2000; 95: 999-1007.

[11] Whitehead WE, Bosmajian L, Zonderman AB, Costa PT, Shuster MM. Symptoms of psychological distress associated with irritable syndrome. Comparison of community and medical clinical samples. *Gastroenterolog* 1988; 95: 709-714.

[12] Fowlie S, Eastwood MA, Ford MJ. Irritable bowel syndrome: the influence of psychological factors on the symptom complex. *J Psychosom Res* 1992; 36: 169-173.

[13] Thompson WG, Heaton KW, Smyth GT, Smyth C. Irritable bowel syndrome in general practice: prevalence characteristics and referral. *Gut* 2000; 46: 78-82.

[14] Schmulson MJ, Ortiz-Garrido OM, Hinojosa C, Arcila D. A single session of reassurance can acutely improve the self perception of impairment in patients with IBS. *J Psychosom Res* 2006; 6: 461-467.

[15] Clowell LJ, Prather CM, Philips SF, Zinsmeister AR. Effects of an irritable bowel syndrome educational class on health-promoting behaviors and symptoms. *Am J Gastroenterol* 1998; 93: 901-905.

[16] Ringstöm G, Störsud S, Lundqvist S, Westman B, Simrèn M. Development of an educational intervention for patients with irritable

bowel syndrome (IBS)- a pilot study. *BMC Gastroenterology* 2009; 9: 10-18.

[17] Ringstöm G, Störsud S, Posserud I, Lundqvist S, Westman B, Simrèn M. Structured patient education is superior to written information in the management of patients with irritable bowel syndrome: a randomized controlled study. *Eur J Gastroenterol Hepatol* 2010; 22: 420-428.

[18] Gibson PR, Shepherd SJ. Evidence-based dietary management of functional gastrointestinal symptoms: The FODMAP approach. *J Gastroenterol Hepatol* 2010; 25: 252-258.

[19] Ong DK, Mitchell SB, Barrett JS, Shepherd SJ, Irving PM, Biesiekierski JR, Smith S, Gibson PR, Muir JG. Manipulation of dietary short chain carbohydrates alters the pattern of gas production and genesis of symptoms in irritable bowel syndrome. *J Gastroenterol Hepatol* 2010; 25:1366-1373.

[20] Zuckerman MJ. The role of fiber in the treatment of irritable bowel syndrome: therapeutic recommendations. *J Clin Gastroenterol* 2006; 40:104-108.

[21] Francis CY, Whorwell PJ. Bran and irritable bowel syndrome: time for reappraisal. *Lancet* 1994; 344: 39-40.

[22] Hebden JM, Blackshaw E, D'Amato M, Perkins AC, Spiller RC. Abnormalities of GI transit in bloated irritable bowel syndrome: effect of bran on transit and symptoms. *Am J Gastroenterol* 2002; 97: 2315-2320.

[23] Aller R, de Luis DA, Izaola O, la Calle F, del Olmo L, Fernandez L, Arranz T, González Hernandez JM. Effects of a high-fiber diet on symptoms of irritable bowel syndrome: a randomized clinical trial. *Nutrition* 2004; 20: 735-737.

[24] Heizer WD, Southern S, McGovern S. The role of diet in symptoms of irritable bowel syndrome in adults: a narrative review. *J Am Diet Assoc* 2009; 109: 1204-1214.

[25] Paineau D, Payen F, Panserieu S, Coulombier G, Sobaszek A, Lartigau I, Brabet M, Galmiche JP, Tripodi D, Sacher-Huvelin S, Chapalain V, Zourabichvili O, Respondek F, Wagner A, Bornet FR.The effects of regular consumption of short-chain fructo-oligosaccharides on digestive comfort of subjects with minor functional bowel disorders. *Br J Nutr* 2008; 99: 311-318.

[26] Østgaard H, Hausken T, Gundersen D, El-Salhy M. Diet and effects of diet management on quality of life and symptoms in patients with irritable bowel syndrome. *Mol Med Rep* in press.

[27] Levy RL, Linde JA, Feld KA, Crowell MD, Jeffery RW. The association of gastrointestinal symptoms with weight diet and exercise in weight-loss program participants. *Clin Gastroenterol Hepatol* 2005; 2: 992-996.

[28] Daley AJ, Grimmett C, Roberts L, Wilson S, Fatek M, Roalfe A, Singh S. The effects of exercise upon symptoms and quality of life in patients diagnosed with irritable bowel syndrome: a randomised controlled trial. *Int J Sports Med* 2008; 29: 778-782.

[29] Johannesson E, Simrèn M, Strid H, Bajor A, Sadik R. Physical activity improves symptoms in irritable bowel syndrome: a randomized controlled trial. *Am J Gastroenterol* 2011; 106: 915-922.

[30] Chey WD, Rai J. Exercise and IBS: no pain, no gain. *Gastroenterology* 2011; 141: 1941-1943.

[31] Strid H, Simrèn M, Störsund S, Stotzer PO, Sadik R.Effect of heavy exercise on gastrointestinal transit in edurance athletes. *Scand J Gatroenterol* 2011; 46: 673-677.

[32] Wang Y, Kondo T, Suzukamo Y, Oouchida Y, Izumi S. Vagal nerve regulation is essential for the increase in gastric motility in response to mild exercise. Tohoku *J Exp Med* 2010; 222: 155-163.

[33] Rehrer NJ, Beckers EJ, Brouns F, Saris WH, Ten Hoor F. Effects of electrolytes in carbohydrate beverages on gastric emptying and secretion. *Med Sci Sports Exerc* 1993; 25: 42-51.

[34] Food and agriculture Organization on the UN and World Health Organization Working Group. Guidelines for the evaluation of probiotics in food. Rome/Geneva: FAO/WHO; 2002.

[35] Whelan K. Probiotics and prebiotics in the management of irritable bowel syndromr. a review of recent clinical trials and systematic reviews. *Curr Opin nutr Metab Care* 2011; 14: 581-587.

[36] Whorell PJ. Do probiotics improve symptoms in patients with irritable bowel syndrome? *Ther Adv Gastroenterol* 2009; 2 (Suppl 1); s37-s44.

[37] Spiller R. Review article: probiotics and prebiotics in irritable bowel syndrome. *Aliment Pharmacol Ther* 2008; 28: 385-396.

[38] Nobaek S, Johansson ML, Molin G, Ahrne S, Jeppsson. Alteration of intestinal microflora is associated with reduction in abdominal bloating and pain in patients with irritable bowel syndrome. *Am J Gastroenterol* 2000; 95: 1231-1238.

[39] Niedzielin K, Kordecki H, Birkenfeld B. A controlled, double-blind, randomized study on the efficacy of *Lactobacillus plantrum* 299v in patients with irritable bowel syndrome. *Eur J Gastroenterol Hepatol* 2001; 13: 1143-1147.

[40] Sen S, Mullan MM, parker TJ, Woolner JT, Tarry SA, Hunter JO. Effect of *Lactobacillus plantrum* 299v on colonic fermentation and symptoms of irritable bowel syndrome. *Dig Dis Sci* 2002; 47: 2615-2620.

[41] O'Sullivan MA, O'Morain CA. Bacterial supplementation in the irritable bowel syndrome. A randomised double-blind placebo controlled crossover study. *Dig Liver Dis* 2000; 32: 294-301.

[42] Bauserman M, Michail S. The use of *lactobacillus GG* irritable bowel syndrome in children: a double-blind randomized control trial. *J Pediatr* 2005; 147: 197-201.

[43] Gawronska A, Dziechciarz P, Horvath A, Szajewska H. A randomized double-blind placebo-controlled trial of *Lactobacillus GG* for abdominal pain disorders in children. *Aliment Pharmacol Ther* 2007; 25: 177-184.

[44] Niv E, Naftali T, Hallak R, Vaisman N. The efficacy of *Lactobacillus reuteri* ATCC 55730 in the treatment of patients with irritable bowel syndrome -a double blind, placebo-controlled, randomized study. *Clin Nutr* 2005; 24: 925-931.

[45] Halpern GM, Prindiville T, Blankebburg M, Hsia T, Gershwin ME. Treatment of irritable bowel syndrome with lacteol fort: arandomized, double-blind, cross-over trial. *Am J Gastroenterol* 1996; 91: 1579-1585.

[46] Gade J, Thorn P. Paraghurt for patients with irritable bowel syndrome. A controlled clinical investigation from general practice. *Scan J Prim Health Care* 1989; 7: 23-26.

[47] Guyonnet D, Chassany O, Ducortte P, Picard C, Mouret M, Mercier CH, Matuchansky C. Effect of a fermented milk containing *Bifidobacterium animalis* DN-173 010 on health-related quality of life and symptoms in irritable bowel syndrome in adults in primary care: a multicenre , randomized, double-blind, controlled trial. *Aliment Pharmacol Ther* 2007; 26: 475-486.

[48] Kim HJ, Camilleri M, Mckinzie S, Lempke MB, Burton DD, Thomforde GM, Zinsmeister AR. A randomized controlled trial of a probiotic, VSL#3, on a gut transit and symptom in diahrrhoea-predominant irritable bowel syndrome. *Aliment Pharmacol Ther* 2003; 17: 895-904.

[49] Kim HJ, Vazquez Roque MI, Camilleri M, Stephens D, Burton DD, Baxter K, Thomforde G, Zinsmeister AR. A randomized controlled trial of a probiotic combination VSL#3 and placebo in irritable bowel syndrome. with bloating. *Neurogastroenterol Motil* 2005; 17: 687-696.

[50] Kajander K, Hatakka K, Poussa T, Farkkila M, Korpela R. A probiotic mixture alleviates symptoms in irritable bowel syndrome patients: a

controlled 6-month intervention. *Aliment Pharmacol Ther* 2005; 22: 387-394.

[51] Kajander K, Myllyluoma E, Rajilić-Stojanović M, Kyrönpalo S, Rasmussen M, Järvenpää S, Zoetendal EG, de Vos WM, Vapaatalo H, Korpela R. Clinical trial: multispecies probiotic supplementation alleviates the symptoms of irritable bowel syndrome and stabilizes intestinal microbiota. *Aliment Pharmacol Ther* 2008; 27: 48-57.

[52] Drouault-Holowacz S, Bieuvelet S, Burckel A, Cazaubiel M, Dray X, Marteau P. A double blind randomized controlled trial of probiotic combination in 100 patients with irritable bowel syndrome. *Gastroenterol Clin Biol* 2008; 32: 147-152.

[53] Enck P, Zimmerman K, Menke G, Muller-Lissner S, Martens U, Klosterhalften S. A mixture of *Escherichia coli* (DSM 17252) and *Enterococus Faecalis* (DSM 16440) for teatment of the irritable bowel syndrome- a randomized controlled trial with primary care physicians. *Neurogastroenterol Motil* 2008; 20: 1103-1109.

[54] Aragon G, Graham DB, Doman DB. Probiotic therapy for irritable bowel syndrome. *Gastroenterol Hepatol* 2010; 6: 39-44.

[55] El-Salhy M, Lillebø E, Reinemo A, Salmelid L, Hausken T. Effects of a health program comprising reassurance, diet management, probiotic administration and regular exercise on symptoms and quality of life in patients with irritable bowel syndrome. *Gastroenterology Insights* 2010; 2: 21-26.

[56] Shen D, Zhu Y, Lu J. Polymerase chain reaction of *Lactobacillus* acidophilus in human oral cavity and fecal samles after 2-week consumption of yoghurt. *Acta Odontol Scand* 2010; 69: 27-32.

[57] Roberfroid M, Gibson GR, Hoyles L, McCartney AL, Rastall R, Rowland I, Wolvers D, Watzl B, Szajewska H, Stahl B, Guarner F, Respondek F, Whelan K, Coxam V, Davicco MJ, Léotoing L, Wittrant Y, Delzenne NM, Cani PD, Neyrinck AM, Meheust A. Prebiotics effects: metabolic and health benefits. *Br J Nutr* 2010; 104 (Suppl 2): S1-S63.

[58] Whorwell PJ, Prior A, Faragher EB. Controlled trial of hypnotherapy in the treatment of severe refractory irritable bowel syndrome. *Lancet* 1984; 2: 1232-1234.

[59] Palsson OS, Turner MJ, Johnson DA, Burnelt CK, Whitehead WE. Hypnosis treatment for severe irritable bowel syndrome: investigation of mechanisms and effects on symptoms. *Dig Dis* Sci 2002; 47: 2605-2615.

[60] Lindfors P, Unge P, Arvidsson P, Nyhlin H, Björnsson E, Abrahammsson H, Simrèn M. Effects of gut-directed hypnotherapy on IBS in different clinical settings-results from two randomized, controlled trials. *Am J Gastroenterol* 2011; doi:10.1038/ajg.2011.340.

[61] Wilson S, Maddison T, Roberts L, Greenfield S, Singh S. Systemic review: the effectiveness of hypnotherapy in the management of irritable bowel syndrome. *Aliment Pharmacol Ther* 2006; 24: 769-780.

[62] Palsson O, Turner M, Whitehead W. Hypnosis home treatment for irritable bowel syndrome: a pilot Study. *Int J Clin Exp Hypn* 2006; 54: 85-99.

[63] Gonsalkorale VM, Haughton LA, Whorwell PJ. Hypnotherapy in irritable bowel syndrome: a large-scale audit of a clinical service with examination of factors influencing responsiveness. *Am J Gatroenterol* 2002; 97: 954-961.

[64] Tan G, Hammond DC, Gurrala J. Hypnosis and irritable bowel syndrome: A review of efficacy and mechanism of action. *Am J Clin Hypnosis* 2005; 47: 161-178.

[65] Whorwell PJ. Effective management of irritable bowel syndrome-the Manchester model. *Int J Clin Exp Hypnosis* 2006; 54: 21-26.

[66] Lea R, Houghton LA, Calvert EL, Larder S, Gonsalkorale WM, Whelan V, Randles J, Cooper P, Cruickshanks P, Miller V, Whorwell PJ. Gut-focused hypnotherapy normalises disordered rectal sensitivity in patients with irritable bowel syndrome. *Aliment Pharmacol Ther* 2003; 17: 635-642.

[67] Whorwe PJ, Houghton LA, Taylor EE, Maxton DG. Physiological effects of emotion: Assessment via hypnosis. *Lancet* 1992; 340: 69-72.

[68] Rainville P, Duncan GH, Price DD, Carrier B, Bushnell MC. Pain affect encoded in human anterior cingulate but not somatosensory cortex. *Science* 1997; 277: 968-971.

[69] Kennedy T, Jones R, Darnley S, Seed P, Wessely S, Chalder T.Cognitive behaviour therapy in addition to antispasmodic treatment for irritable bowel syndrome in primary care: randomised controlled trial. *BMJ* 2005; 331: 435-440.

[70] Payne A, Blanchard EB. A controlled comparison of cognitive therapy and selfhelp support groups in the treatment of irritable bowel syndrome. *J Consult Clin Psychol* 1995; 63: 779–786.

[71] Drossman DA, Toner BB, Whitehead WE, Diamant NE, Dalton CB, Duncan S, Emmott S, Proffitt V, Akman D, Frusciante K, Le T, Meyer K, Bradshaw B, Mikula K, Morris CB, Blackman CJ, Hu Y, Jia H, Li

JZ, Koch GG, Bangdiwala SI. Cognitive-behavioral therapyversus education and desipramine versus placebo for moderate to severefunctional bowel disorders. *Gastroenterology* 2003; 125: 19–31.

[72] Van Dulmen AM, Fennis JM, Bleijenberg G. Cognitive-behavioral grouptherapy for irritable bowel syndrome: Effects and long-term follow-up.*Psychosom Med* 1996; 58: 508–514.

[73] Lackner JM, Jaccard J, Krasner SS, Katz LA, Gudeski GD, Blanchard EB. How does congnitive behavior therapy for IBS work?: A mediational analysis of a randomized clinical trial. *Gastroenterology* 2007; 133: 433-444.

[74] Jones M, Koloski N, Boyce P, Talley NJ. Pathways concerning cognitive behavioral therapy and change in bowel symptoms of IBS. *J Psychosom Res* 2011; 70: 278-275.

[75] Guthrie E. Brief psychotherapy with patients with refractory irritable bowel syndrome. *Br J Psychother* 1991; 8: 175-188.

[76] Guthrie E, Creed F, Dawson D, Tomenson B. A controlled trial of psychological treatment for the irritable bowel syndrome. *Gastroenterology* 1991; 100: 450–457.

[77] Svedlund J, Sjodin I, Ottosson J, Dotevall G. Controlled study of psychotherapy in irritable bowel syndrome. Lancet, 1983; ii: 589-592.

[78] Creed F, Fernandes L, Guthrie E, Palmer S, Ratcliffe J, Read N, Rigby C, Thompson D, Tomenson B; North of England IBS Research Group. The cost-effectiveness of psychotherapy and paroxetine for severe irritable bowel syndrome. *Gastroenterology* 2003; 124: 303-317.

[79] Blanchard EB, Schwarz SP, Neff DF, Gerardi MA. Prediction of outcome from the selfregulatory treatment of irritable bowel syndrome. *Behav Res Ther* 1988; 26: 187-190.

[80] Neff DF, Blachard EB. A multi-component treatment for irritable bowel syndrome. *Behav Ther* 1987; 18: 70-83.

[81] Lynch PM, Zamble E. A controlled behavioral treatment study of irritable bowel syndrome. *Behav Ther* 1989; 20: 509-523.

[82] Blanchard EB, Greene B, Scharff L, Schwarz-McMorris SP. Relaxation training as a treatment for irritable bowel syndrome. *Biofeedback Self Regul* 1993; 18: 125-132.

[83] Voirol MW, Hipolito J. Relaxation in the treatment of irritable gut: Results after 40 months. *Schweiz Med Wochenschr* 1987; 117: 1117–1119.

[84] Khan S, Chang L. Diagnosis and management of IBS. *Nat Rev Gastroenterol Hepatol* 2010; 7: 565-581.

[85] Spiller RC. Treatment of irritable bowel syndrome. *Curr Options Gastroenterol* 2003; 6: 329-337.

[86] Lacy BE, Weiser K, De Lee R. The treatment of irritable bowel syndrome. *Ther Adv Gastroenterol* 2009; 2: 221-238.

[87] Schmulson M, Chang L. Review article: the treatment of functional bloating and distension. *Aliment Pharmacol Ther* 2011; 33: 1071-1086.

[88] Cann PA, Read NW, Holdsworth CD, Barends D. Role of loperamide and placebo in management of irritable bowel syndrome (IBS). *Dig Dis Sci* 1984; 29: 239-247

[89] Lavo B, Stenstam M, Nielsen A-L. Loperamide in treatment of irritable bowel syndrome - A double-blind placebo controlled study. *Scand J Gastroenterol Suppl* 1987; 22: 77-80.

[90] McQuay HJ, Tramer M, Nye BA, Carroll D, Wiffen PJ, Moore RA. A systematic review of antidepressants in neuropathic pain. *Pain* 1996; 68: 217-227.

[91] Mertz H, Fass R, Kodner A, Yan-Go F, Fullerton S, Mayer EA. Effect of amitriptyline on symptoms, sleep, and visceral perception in patients with functional dyspepsia. *Am J Gastroenterol* 1998; 93: 160-165.

[92] Clouse RE, Lustman PJ. Use of psychopharmacological agents for functional gastrointestinal disorders. Gut 2005; 54: 1332-1341.

[93] Grover M, Drossman DA. Psychotrofic agents in functional gastrointestinal disorders. *Curr Opin Pharmacol* 2008; 8: 715-723.

[94] Tack J, Broekaert D, Fischler B, Van Oudenhove L, Gevers AM, Janssens J. A controlled crossover study of the selective serotonin reuptake inhibitor citalopram in irritable bowel syndrome. *Gut* 2006; 55: 1095–1103.

[95] Creed F, Fernandes L, Guthrie E, Palmer S, Ratcliffe J, Read N, Rigby C, Thompson D, Tomenson B; North of England IBS Research Group. The cost-effectiveness of psychotherapy and paroxetine for severe irritable bowel syndrome. *Gastroenterology* 2003; 124: 303-317.

[96] Kuiken SD, Tytgat GN, Boeckxstaens GE. The selective serotonin reuptake inhibitor fluoxetine does not change rectal sensitivity and symptoms in patients with irritable bowel syndrome: a double blind, randomized, placebo-controlled study. *Clin Gastroenterol Hepatol* 2003; 1: 219-228.

[97] Tabas G, Beaves M, Wang J, Friday P, Mardini H, Arnold G. Paroxetine to treat irritable bowel syndrome not responding to high-fiber diet: a double-blind, placebo-controlled trial. *Am J Gastroenterol* 2004; 99: 914-920.

[98] Frissora CL, Cash BD. Review article: the role of antibiotics vs. conventional pharmacotherapy in treating symptoms of irritable bowel syndrome. *Aliment Pharmacol Ther* 2007; 25: 1271-1281.

[99] Ducrottè P. Irritable bowel syndrome: dietary and pharmacological therapeutic options. *Gastroenterol Clin Biol* 2009; 33 Suppl 1: S68-78.

[100] Pimentel M, Chatterjee S, Chow EJ, Park S, Kong Y. Neomycin improves constipation-predominant irritable bowel syndrome in a fashion that is dependent on the prescence of methane gas: subanalysis of a double-blind randomized controlled study. *Dig Dis Sci* 2006; 51: 1297-1301.

[101] Shara A, Aoun E, Adul-Baki H, Mounzer R, Sidani S, Elhaji I. A randomized double-blind placebo-controlled trial of rifaximin in patients with adominal bloating and flatulence. *Am J Gastroenterol* 2006; 10: 326-333.

[102] Fumi AL, Trexier K. Rifaximin treatment for symptoms of irritable bowel syndrome. *Ann Pharmacother* 2008; 42: 408-412.

[103] Pimentel M, Park S, Mirocha J, Kane SV, Kong Y. The effect of nonabsorbed oral antibiotic (rifaximin) on the symptoms of the irritable bowel syndrome: a randomized trial. *Ann Intern Med* 2006; 145: 557-563.

[104] Pimentel M. Review of ifaximin as treatment for SIBO and IBS. Expert Opin Investig Drugs 2009; 18: 349-358.

[105] Ford AC, Talley NJ, Spiegel BM, Foxx-Orenstein AE, Schiller L, Quigley EM, Moayyedi P. Effect of fibre, antispasmodics, and peppermint oil in the treatment of irritable bowel syndrome: systematic review and meta-analysis. *BMJ* 2008; 337: a2313.

[106] Bijkerk CJ, de Wit NJ, Muris JW, Whorwell PJ, Knottnerus JA, Hoes AW. Soluble or insoluble fibre in irritable bowel syndrome in primary care? Randomised placebo controlled trial. *BMJ* 2009; 339: b3154.

[107] Snook J, Shepherd HA. Brain supplementation in the treatment of irritable bowel syndrome. *Aliment Pharmacol Ther* 1997; 8: 511-514.

[108] Prior A, Whorwell PJ. Double blind study of ispaghula in irritable bowel syndrome. *Gut* 1987; 28: 1510-1513.

[109] Award RA, Camacho S. A randomized double-blind, placebo-controlled trial of polethylene glycol effects on fasting and postprandial rectal sensitivity and symptoms in hypersensitive constipation-predominant irritable bowel syndrome. *Colorectal Dis* 2009; 12: 1131-1138.

[110] Klein K B. Controlled treatment trials in the irritable bowel syndrome: a critical appraisal. *Gastroenterology* 1988. 95: 232-241.

[111] Poynard T, Naveau S, Mory B, Chaput JC. Meta-analysis of smooth muscle relaxants in the treatment of irritable bowel syndrome. *Aliment Pharmacol Ther* 1994; 8499-8510.

[112] Jailwala J, Imperiale T F, Kroenke K. Pharmacologic treatment of the irritable bowel syndrome: a systematic review of randomized, controlled trials. *Ann Intern Med* 2000; 13: 3136-3147.

[113] Poynard T, Regimbeau C, Benhamou Y. Meta-analysis of smooth muscle relaxants in the treatment of irritable bowel syndrome. *Aliment Pharmacol Ther* 2001; 15: 355–361.

[114] Song GH, Leng PH, Gwee KA, Moochhala SM, Ho KY. Melatonin improves abdominal pain in irritable bowel syndrome patients who have slep disturbances: a randomised, double blind, placebo controlled study. *Gut* 2005; 54: 1402-1407.

[115] Lu WZ, Gwee KA, Moochhala SM, Ho KY.Melatonin improves bowel symptoms in female patients with irritable bowel syndrome: a double blind, placebo controlled study. *Allment Pharmacol Ther* 2005; 22: 927-934.

[116] Kim D-Y, Camilleri M. Serotonin: a mediator of the brain-gut connection. *Am J Gastroenterol* 2000; 95: 2698-2709.

[117] Barnes NM, Sharp T. A review of central 5-HT receptors and their function. *Neuropharmacology* 1999; 38: 1083-1152.

[118] Talley NJ. 5-Hydroxytryptamine agonists and antagonists in the modulation of gastrointestinal motility and sensation: clinical implications. *Aliment Pharmacol Ther* 1992; 6: 273-289.

[119] Tack J, Demedts I, Dehondt G, Caenepeel P, Fischler B, Zandecki M, Janssens J. Clinical and pathophysiological characteristics of acute-onset functional dyspepsia. *Gastroenterology* 2002; 122: 1738-1747.

[120] Tack JF, Janssens J, Vantrappen G, Wood JD. Actions of 5-hydroxytryptamine on myenteric neurones in the gastric antrum of the guinea pig. *Am J Physiol* 1992; 263: G838–G846.

[121] Coulie B, Tack J, Maes B, Geypens B, De Roo M, Jensens J. Sumatriptan, a selective 5-HT 1 receptor agonist, induces a lag phase for gastric emptying of liquids in humans. *Am J Physiol* 1997; 272: G902-G908.

[122] Hillsley K, Kirkup AJ, Grundy D. Direct and indirect actions of 5-hydroxytryptamine on the discharge of mesenteric afferent fibers innervating the rat jejunum. *J Physiol* (Lond) 1998; 506: 551–561.

[123] Tack J, Vanden Berghe P, Coulie B, Janssens J. Sumatriptan is an agonist at 5-HT1P receptors on myenteric neurones in the guinea pig gastric antrum. *Neurogastroenterol Motil* 2007; 19: 39-46.

[124] Tack J, Coulie B, Wilmer A, Peeters T, Janssens J. Actions of the 5-hydroxytryptamine-1 receptor agonist sumatriptan on interdigestive gastrointestinal motility in human. *Gut* 1998; 42: 36-41.

[125] Tack J, Piessevaux H, Coulie B, Fischler B, De Gucht V, Janssens J. A placebo-controlled trial of buspirone, a fundus relaxing drug in functional dyspepsia: effect on symptoms and gastric sensory motor function. (abstr) *Gastroenterology* 1999; 116: A325.

[126] Tack J, Van Den Elzen B, Tytgat G, Wajs E, Van Nueten V L, De Ridder F, Boeckxstaens G. A placebo-controlled trial of the 5-HT1A agonist R-137696 on symptoms, visceral hypersensitivity and on impaired accommodation in functional dyspepsia. (abstr) *Gastroenterology* 2004; 126: A70.

[127] Tack J, Piessevaux H, Coulie B, Caenepeel P, Janssens J. Role of impaired gastric accommodation to a meal in functional dyspepsia. *Gastroenterology* 1998; 115: 1346-1352.

[128] Tack J, Caenepeel P, Corsetti M, Janssens J. Role of tension receptors in dyspeptic patients with hypersensitivity to gastric distention. *Gastroenterology* 2004; 127: 1058-1066.

[129] Gershon MD, Tack J. The serotonin signaling system: from basic understanding to drug development for functional GI disorders. *Gastroenterology* 2007; 132: 397-414.

[130] Hammer J, Phillips SF, Talley NJ, Camilleri M. Effect of a 5HT3-antagonist (ondansetron) on rectal sensitivity and compliance in health and the irritable bowel syndrome. *Aliment Pharmacol Ther* 1993; 7: 543–551.

[131] Zerbib F, Bruley des Varannes S, Oriola RC, McDonald J, Isal JP, Galmiche JP. Aldosterone does not affect the visceral perception of gastric distension in healthy subjects. *Aliment Pharmacol Ther* 1994; 8: 403-407.

[132] Zighelboim J, Talley NJ, Phillips SF, Harmsen WS, Zinsmeister AR. Visceral perception in irritable bowel syndrome (Rectal and gastric responses to distension and serotonin type 3 antagonism). *Dig Dis Sci* 1995; 40: 819-827.

[133] Ladabaum U, Brown MB, Pan W, Owyang C, Hasler WL. Effects of nutrients and serotonin 5-HT3 antagonism on symptoms evoked by

distal gastric distension in humans. *Am J Physiol Gastrointest Liver Physiol* 2001; 280: G201-G208.

[134] Delvaux M, Louvel D, Mamet JP, Campos-Oriola R, Frexinos J. Effect of aldosterone on responses to colonic distension in patients with irritable bowel syndrome. *Aliment Pharmacol Ther* 1998; 12: 849-855.

[135] Feinle C, Read NW. Ondansetron reduces nausea induced by gastroduodenal stimulation without changing gastric motility. *Am J Physiol* 1006; 271: G591–G597.

[136] Simren M, Simms L, D'Souza D, Abrahamsson H, Bjornsson ES. Lipid-induced colonic hypersensitivity in irritable bowel syndrome: the role of 5-HT3 receptors. *Aliment Pharmacol Ther* 2003; 17: 279-287.

[137] Jones RH, Holtmann G, Rodrigo L, Ehsanullah RS, Crompton PM, Jacques LA, Mills JG. Alosetron relieves pain and Improves bowel function compared with mebeverine in female in nonconstipated irritable bowel syndrome patients. *Aliment Pharmacol Ther* 1999; 13: 1419-1427.

[138] Camilleri M, Mayer EA, Drossman DA, Heath A, Dukes GE, McSorley D, Kong S, Mangel AW, Northcutt AR. Improvement in pain and bowel function in female irritable bowel patients with alosetron, a 5-HT3 receptor antagonist. *Aliment Pharmacol Ther* 1999; 13: 1149-1159.

[139] Camilleri M, Northcutt AR, Kong SA, Dukes GE, McSorley D, Mangel AM. Efficacy and safety of alosetron in women with irritable bowel syndrome: a randomised, placebo-controlled trial. *Lancet* 2000; 355: 1035-1040.

[140] Bardhan KD, Bodemar G, Geldof H, Schütz E, Heath A, Mills JG, Jacques LA. A double-blind, randomized, placebo-controlled dose-ranging study to evaluate the efficacy of alosetron in the treatment of irritable bowel syndrome. *Aliment Pharmacol Ther* 2000; 14: 23-34.

[141] Lembo T, Wright RA, Bagby B, Ecker DC, Ordon GS, Jhingran P, Carter E, Lotronex Investigator Team. Alosetron controls bowel urgency and provides global symptom improvement in women with diarrhea-predominant irritable bowel syndrome. *Am J Gastroenterol* 2001; 96: 2662-2670.

[142] Thompson CA. Alosetron withdrawn from market. *Am J Health Syst Pharm* 2001; 58: 13.

[143] Chey WD, Cash BD. Cilansetron: a new serotonergic agent for the irritable bowel syndrome with diarrhoea. *Expert Opin Investig Drugs* 2005; 14: 185-193.

[144] Talley NJ, Van Zanten SV, Saez LR, Dukes G, Perschy T, Heath M, Leoudis KC, Mangel AW. Heath M: A dose-ranging, placebo-controlled, randomized trial of alosetron in patients with functional dyspepsia. *Aliment Pharmacol Ther* 2001; 15: 525-537.

[145] Furness JB, Kunze WA, Clerc N. Nutrient tasting and signalling mechanisms in the gut II. The intestine as a sensory organ: neural, endocrine, and immune response. *Am J Physiol* 1999; 277: G922-G928.

[146] Tuladhar BR, Costall B, Naylor RJ. 5-HT 3 and 5-HT 4 receptor-mediated facilitation of the emptying phase of the peristaltic reflex in the marmoset isolated ileum. *Br J Phamacol* 1996; 117: 1679-1684.

[147] Prins NH, Akkermans IM, Lefebvre RA, Schuurkes JA. 5-HT 4 receptors on cholinergic nerves involved in contractility of canine and human large intestine longitudinal muscle. *Br J* Phamacol 2000; 131: 927-932.

[148] Grider JR, Foxx-Orenstein AE, Jin JG. 5-Hydroxytryptamine 4 receptor agonists initiate the peristaltic reflex in human, rat and guinea pig intestines. *Gastroenterology* 1998; 5: 370-380.

[149] Tarn FS, Illier HK, Bunce KT. Characterization of the 5-hydroxytryptamine receptor type involved in inhibition of spontaneous activity of human isolated colonic circular muscle. *Br J Phamacol* 1994; 113: 143-150.

[150] Hillier K, Tarn FS-F, Bunce KT, Grossman C. Inhibition of motility induced by the activation of 5-HTI-like and 5-HT4-like receptors in isolated human colon smooth muscle. *Br J Phamacol* 1994; 112: 102P.

[151] Borman RA, Burleigh DE. Human colonic mucosa possesses a mixed population of 5-hydroxytrypamine receptors. *Eur J Phamacol* 1996; 309: 271-274.

[152] Prather CM, Camilleri M, Zinsmeister AR, McKinzie S, Thomforde S. Tegaserod accelerates orocecal transit in patients with constipation-predominant irritable bowel syndrome. *Gastroenterology* 2000; 118: 462–468.

[153] Coleski R, Owyang C, Hasler WL. Modulation of intestinal gas dynamics in healthy human volunteers by the 5-HT receptor agonist tegaserod. *Am J Gastroenterol* 2006; 101: 1858–1865.

[154] Pasricha PJ. Desperately seeking serotonin: a commentary on the withdrawal of tegaserod and the state of functional and motility disorders. *Gastroenterology* 2007; 132: 2287-2290.

[155] Bouras EP, Camilleri M, Burton DD, Thomforde G, McKinzie S, Zinsmeister AR. Prucalopride accelerates gastrointestinal and colonic

transit in patients with constipation without a rectal evacuation disorder. *Gastroenterology* 12001; 20: 354–360.

[156] Spiller RC, Trotman IF, Higgins BE, Ghatei MA, Grimble GK, Lee YC, Bloom SR, Misiewicz JJ, Silk DB. The ileal brake-inhibition of jejunal motility after ileal fat perfusion in man. *Gut* 1984; 25: 365–374.

[157] El-Salhy M, Lillebø E, Reinemo A, Salmelid L, Hausken T. Effects of a health program comprising reassurance, diet management, probiotics and regular exercise on symptoms and quality of life in patients with irritable bowel syndrome. *Gastroenterology Insights* 2010; 2: 21-26.

[158] El-Salhy M, Østgaard H, Gundersen D, Hatlebakk JG, Hausken T. The role of diet in the pathogenesis and management of irritable bowel syndrome. *Int J Mol Med* 2012; 29: 723-731.

[159] Østgaard H, Hausken T, Gundersen D, El-Salhy M. Diet and effects of diet management on quality of life and symptoms in patients with irritable bowel syndrome. *Mol Med Rep*, 2012; 5: 1382-1390.

[160] Kaptchuk TJ. Acupuncture: theory, efficacy, and practice. *Ann Intern Med* 2002; 136: 374-383.

[161] Xiao WB, Liu Yl. Rectal hypersensitivity reduced by acupoint TENS in patients with diarrhea-predominant irritable bowel syndrome: a pilot study. *Dig Dis Sci* 2004; 49: 312-319.

[162] Cui KM, Li WM, Gao X, Chung JM, Wu GC. Electro-acupuncutre relieves chronic visceral hyperalgesia in rats. *Neurosci Lett* 2005; 376: 20-23.

[163] Tillisch K. Complementary and alternative medicine for functional gastrointestinal disorders. *Gut* 2006; 55: 593-596.

[164] Reynolds JA, Bland JM, MacPherson H. Acupuncture in irritable bowel syndrome-an exploratory randomized controlled trial. *Acupunct Med* 2008; 26: 8-16.

[165] Lim B, Manheimer E, Lao L, Ziea E, Wisniewski J, Berman B. Acupuncture for treatment of irritable bowel syndrome. *Cochrane Database Sys Rev* 2006 CD005111.

[166] Lembo AJ, Conboy L, Kelley JM, Schnyer RS, McManus C, Quilty MT, Kerr CE, Jacobson EE, Davis RB, Kaptchuk TJ. A treatment trial of acupuncture in IBS patients. *Am J Gastroenterol* 2009; 104: 1489-1497.

[167] Schneider A, Enck P, Streitberger K, Weiland C, Bagheri S, Witte S, Friederich HC, Herzog W, Zipfel S. Acupuncture treatment in irritable bowel syndrome. *Gut* 2006; 55: 649-654.

[168] Wu JCY. Complementary and alternative medicine modalities for the treatment of irritable bowel syndrome: facts or myths? *Gastroenterol Hepatol* 2010; 6: 705-711.

[169] Yoon SL, Grundmann O, Koepp L, Farrell L. Management of irritable bowel syndrome (IBS) in adults: conventional and complementary/alternative approaches. *Altern Med Rev* 2011; 16: 134-151.

[170] Bensoussan Tally NJ, Hing M, Menzies R, Guo A, Ngu M. Treatment of irritable bowel syndrome with Chinese herbal medicine: a randomized controlled trial. *JAMA* 1998; 280: 1585-1589.

[171] Leung WK, Wu JC, Liang SM, Chan LS, Chan FK, Xie H, Fung SS, Hui AJ, Wong VW, Che CT, Sung JJ. Treatment of diarrhea-predominant irritable bowel syndrome with traditional Chinese herbal medicine: a randomized placebo-controlled trial. *Am J Gastroenterol* 2006; 101: 1574-1580.

[172] Sallon S, Ben-Arye E, Davidson R, Shapiro H, Ginsberg G, Ligumsky M. A novel treatment for constipation-predominant irritable bowel syndrome using Padma Lax, a Tibetan herbal formula. *Digestion* 2002; 65:161-171.

[173] Madisch A, Holtmann G, Plein K, Hotz J. Treatment of irritable bowel syndrome with herbal preparations: results of a double-blind, randomized, placebo-controlled, multi-centre trial. *Aliment Pharmacol Ther* 2004; 19: 271-279.

[174] Grigleit HG, Grigoleit P. Pharmacology and preclinical pharmacokinetics of peppermint oil. *Phytomedicine* 2005; 12: 612-616.

[175] Kligler B, Chaudhary S. Peppermint oil. *Am Fam Physician* 2007; 75: 1027-1030.

[176] Pittler MH, Ernst E. Peppermint oil for irritable bowel syndrome: a critical review and meta-analysis. *Am J Gastroenterol* 1998; 93: 1131-1135.

[177] Spanier JA, Howden CW, Jones MP. A systematic review of alternative therapies in the irritable bowel syndrome. *Arch Intern Med* 2003; 163: 265-274.

[178] Cappello G, Spezzaferro M, Grossi L, Manzoli L, Marzio L. Peppermint oil (Mintoil) in the treatment of irritable bowel syndrome: a prospective double-blind placebo-controlled randomized trial. *Dig Liver Dis* 2007; 39: 530-536.

[179] Merat S, Khalili S, Mostajabi P, Ghorbani A, Ansari R, Malekzadeh R. The effect of enteric-coated, delayed-release peppermint oil on irritable bowel syndrome. *Dig Dis* Sci 2010; 55: 1385-1390.

[180] Ford AC, Talley NJ, Spiegel BM, Foxx-Orenstein AE, Schiller L, Quigley EM, Moayyedi P. Effect of fibre, antispasmodics, and peppermint oil in the treatment of irritable bowel syndrome: systematic review and meta-analysis. *BMJ* 2008; 337: a2313.

Chapter VII

Concluding Remarks

Abstract

Irritable bowel syndrome is a common gastrointestinal disorder that represents an economic burden to society due to the high consumption of health-care resources and the non-productivity of IBS patients. IBS patients have a considerably reduced quality of life. The diagnosis of IBS is based on symptom assessment such as Rome III criteria. We believe that it is necessary to combine the Rome III criteria with a physical examination, blood tests, gastroscopy and colonoscopy with biopsies. The pathogenesis of IBS seems to be multifactorial. The following factors play a central role in the pathogenesis of IBS: hereditability and genetics, dietary/intestinal microbiota, low-grade inflammation and disturbances in the neuroendocrine system (NES) of the gut. We proposed the following hypothesis: the cause of IBS is an altered NES. An altered NES would cause abnormal gastrointestinal motility, secretions and sensation. All of such abnormalities are characteristic of IBS. Alterations in the NES could be the result of one or more of the following: genetic factors, dietary intake, intestinal flora or low-grade inflammation. PI-IBS and IBD-IBS represent a considerable subset of IBS. Patients with both PI- and IBD-IBS exhibit low-grade mucosal inflammation and abnormalities in the neuroendocrine system of the gut. The options for the treatment of IBS are non-pharmacological and pharmacological. Most IBS patients show improvement with a combination of non-pharmacological management.

Irritable bowel syndrome is a highly prevalent disorder that considerably reduces patients' quality of life [1-37]. It affects individuals in the most productive phase of their lives.

Irritable bowel syndrome patients consume a considerable amount of health-care resources. Moreover, they represent an economic burden to society in the form of non-productivity and reliance on welfare [38-41].

The diagnosis of IBS is based on symptom assessment such as the Rome criteria. Whereas the latter have been widely used in scientific studies and in gastrointestinal congresses in the past 10 years, they are not, however, used by most clinicians consulted by IBS patients [42-45]. This is not because these clinicians are unaware the Rome criteria, but because of the reality in the clinic. IBS patients that seek a doctor are worried and want to be investigated and are not satisfied by just telling them they fulfil certain criteria. They will repeatedly seek health-care until they are investigated. Some clinicians may be concerned about missing a serious disease, especially when patients are repeatedly admitted to the emergency department with severe abdominal pain. Some eminent gastroenterologists still believe that IBS is an exclusion diagnosis. It was thought that the Rome criteria would save on healthcare resources used in expensive tests and examinations, but this has not been the case (see Chapter 3). We believe that the Rome criteria should be combined with a physical examination, blood tests, gastroscopy, duodenal biopsies and colonoscopy with segmental biopsies. These examinations and tests, in addition to the Rome III criteria, would reassure the patient and exclude coeliac disease, inflammatory bowel disease, microscopic colitis and cancer. Furthermore, performing these examinations and tests would remove the pressure applied by some patients to perform these examinations repeatedly; one can always argue against the need for further investigations if there are no new symptoms. Duodenal chromogranin A cell density seems to be a promising biomarker for the diagnosis of IBS [46].

Historically, patients with IBS presented with gastrointestinal complaints for which physicians could find no organic cause. It is natural and understandable to make comparisons with hysteria, which is also predominant in women. Hysteria has been replaced in modern psychiatry by somatisation disorders and conversion disorders. The notion that IBS is a psychiatric disorder is deeply rooted in clinical practice. This situation was not improved by the huge number of publications on a selected group of IBS patients that showed that IBS patients are more likely to be psychiatrically ill and sexually and/or physically abused than the background population. Many patients with IBS ignore their symptoms and regard them as a normal part of everyday life.

IBS patients with anxiety, depression, somatisation or hypochondriasis are more liable to seek healthcare than other IBS patients. Unless this is borne in mind, incorrect conclusions can be drawn. It is interesting in this context that a hospital-based case control study showed that patients with IBS have a comparable health-related quality of life, level of psychological distress and occurrence of recent stressful life events to age-matched IBD patients [47]. There is no convincing evidence to show that psychological factors play a role in the onset and/or progress of irritable bowel syndrome [48]. The pathogenesis of IBS seems to be multifactorial. There is evidence to show that the following factors play a central role in the pathogenesis of IBS: hereditability and genetics, dietary/intestinal microbiota, low-grade inflammation and disturbances in the neuroendocrine system (NES) of the gut. We propose the following hypothesis: the cause of IBS is an altered NES. An altered NES would cause abnormal gastrointestinal motility, secretions and sensation. Such abnormalities are characteristic of IBS. Alterations in the NES could be the result of one or more of the following: genetic factors, dietary intake, intestinal flora or low-grade inflammation.

Post-infectious IBS [PI-IBS) is the sudden onset of IBS symptoms following gastroenteritis in individuals who have not previously had any gastrointestinal complaints. This subset of IBS represents about 6% to 17% of patients with irritable bowel syndrome. Inflammatory bowel disease associated irritable bowel syndrome (IBD-IBS) is an IBS symptom occurring in inflammatory disease (IBD) patients in remission. IBD-IBS occurs in 33–46% of ulcerative colitis patients, and in 42–60% of Crohn's disease patients in remission. Gastrointestinal infections and possibly non-gastrointestinal infection cause PI-IBS. The prevalence of PI-IBS decreases with time depending on both host- and pathogen-related factors [49-55]. Patients with both PI- and IBD-IBS exhibit low-grade mucosal inflammation and abnormalities in the neuroendocrine system of the gut. The main hormones affected in PI- and IBD-IBS are small intestinal CCK, and large intestinal serotonin and PYY. The pathogenesis of these subsets of IBS is consistent with our proposed hypothesis for the pathogenesis of IBS.

The options for the treatment of IBS are non-pharmacological and pharmacological. The non-pharmacological approach comprises the provision of information, reassurance and dietary guidance, regular exercise, probiotic intake, gut-directed hypnotherapy, cognitive therapy, acupuncture and herbal therapy. Pharmacological treatment depends on the symptoms and mainly includes anti-diarrhoeal drugs, laxatives, antispasmodic drugs, antidepressants, anti-anxiety drugs and antibiotics.

Most IBS patients show improvement with a combination of non-pharmacological management involving information, reassurance, dietary guidance, regular exercise and probiotics. However, depending on the symptoms, some patients also require pharmacological treatment. Loperamide is the first choice for diarrhoea, polyethylene glycol is used for constipation, and peppermint oil and eventually antidepressant are chosen for pain. Few patients with so-called refractory IBS are candidates for gut-directed hypnotherapy.

References

[1]   Quigley EM, Locke GR, Mueller-Lissner S, Paulo LG, Tytgat GN, Helfrich I, Schaefer E. Prevalence and management of abdominal cramping and pain: a multinational survey. *Aliment Pharmacol Ther* 2006; 24: 411-419.

[2]   Vandvik PO, Lydersen S, Farup PG. Prevalence, comorbidity and impact of irritable bowel syndrome in Norway. *Scand J Gastroenterol* 2006; 41: 650-656.

[3]   Drossman DA, Li Z, Andruzzi E, et al. US householder survey of functional gastrointestinal disorders. Prevalence, sociodemography, and health impact. *Dig Dis Sci* 1993; 38: 1569-1580.

[4]   Saito YA, Talley NJ, Melton J, Fett S, Zinsmeister AR, Locke GR. The effect of new diagnostic criteria for irritable bowel syndrome on community prevalence estimates. *Neurogastroenterol Motil* 2003; 15: 687-694.

[5]   Thompson WG, Irvine EJ, Pare P, Ferrazzi S, Rance L. Functional gastrointestinal disorders in Canada: first population-based survey using Rome II criteria with suggestions for improving the questionnaire. *Dig Dis Sci* 2002; 47: 225-235.

[6]   Li FX, Patten SB, Hilsden RJ, Sutherland LR. Irritable bowel syndrome and health-related quality of life: a population-based study in Calgary, Alberta. *Can J Gastroenterol* 2003; 17: 259-263.

[7]   Boyce PM, Koloski NA, Talley NJ. Irritable bowel syndrome according to varying diagnostic criteria: are the new Rome II criteria unnecessarily restrictive for research and practice? *Am J Gastroenterol* 2000; 95: 3176-3183.

[8] Barbezat G, Poulton R, Milne B, Howell S, Fawcett JP, Talley N. Prevalence and correlates of irritable bowel symptoms in a New Zealand birth cohort. *NZ Med J* 2002; 115: U220.

[9] Boekema PJ, van Dam van Isselt EF, Bots ML, Smout AJ. Functional bowel symptoms in a general Dutch population and associations with common stimulants. *Neth J Med* 2001; 59: 23-30.

[10] Mearin F, Badia X, Balboa A, Baró E, Caldwell E, Cucala M, Díaz-Rubio M, Fueyo A, Ponce J, Roset M, Talley NJ. Irritable bowel syndrome prevalence varies enormously depending on the employed diagnostic criteria: comparison of Rome II versus previous criteria in a general population. *Scand J Gastroenterol* 2001; 36: 1155-1161.

[11] Gaburri M, Bassotti G, Bacci G, Cinti A, Bosso R, Ceccarelli P, Paolocci N, Pelli MA, Morelli A. Functional gut disorders and health care seeking behavior in an Italian non-patient population. *Recenti Prog Med* 1989; 80: 241-244.

[12] Coffin B, Dapoigny M, Cloarec D, Comet D, Dyard F. Relationship between severity of symptoms and quality of life in 858 patients with irritable bowel syndrome. *Gastroenterol Clin Biol* 2004; 28: 11-15.

[13] Agreus L, Svarsudd K, Nygren O, Tibblin G. Irritable bowel syndrome and dyspepsia in general population: overlap and lack of stability over time. *Gastroenterology* 1995; 109: 671-680.

[14] Hillila MT, Farkkila MA. Prevalence of irritable bowel syndrome according to different diagnostic criteria in a non-selected adult population. *Aliment Pharmacol Ther* 2004; 20: 339-345.

[15] Kay L, Jorgensen T, Jensen KH. The epidemiology of irritable bowel syndrome in a random population: prevalence, incidence, natural history and risk factors. *J Intern Med* 1994; 236: 23-30.

[16] Hoseini-Asl MK, Amra B. Prevalence of irritable bowel syndrome in Shahrekord, Iran. *Indian J Gastroenterol* 2003; 22: 215-216.

[17] Karaman N, Turkay C, Yonem O. Irritable bowel syndrome prevalence in city center of Sivas. *Turk J Gastroenterol* 2003; 14: 128-131.

[18] Celebi S, Acik Y, Deveci SE, et al. Epidemiological features of irritable bowel syndrome in a Turkish urban society. *J Gastroenterol Hepatol* 2004; 19: 738-743.

[19] Masud MA, Hasan M, Khan AK. Irritable bowel syndrome in a rural community in Bangladesh: prevalence, symptoms pattern, and health care seeking behavior. *Am J Gastroenterol* 2001; 96: 1547-5152.

[20] Huerta I, Valdovinos MA, Schmulson M. Irritable bowel syndrome in Mexico. *Dig Dis* 2001; 19: 251-257.

[21] Kwan AC, Hu WH, Chan YK, et al. Prevalence of irritable bowel syndrome in Hong Kong. *J Gastroenterol Hepatol* 2002; 17: 1180-1186.

[22] Lau EM, Chan FK, Ziea ET, et al. Epidemiology of irritable bowel syndrome in Chinese. *Dig Dis Sci* 2002; 47: 2621-2624.

[23] Schlemper R, Van der Werf SJ, Vandenbroucke JP, et al. Peptic ulcer, non-ulcer dyspepsia and irritable bowel syndrome in The Netherlands and Japan. *Scand J Gastroenterol Suppl* 1993; 28: 33-41.

[24] Ho KY, Kang JY, Seow A. Prevalence of gastrointestinal symptoms in a multiracial Asian population, with particular reference to reflux-type symptoms. *Am J Gastroenterol* 1998; 93: 1816-1822.

[25] Xiong LS, Chen MH, Chen HX, et al. A population-based epidemiologic study of irritable bowel syndrome in South China: stratified randomized study by cluster's sampling. *Aliment Pharmacol Ther* 2004; 19: 1217-1224.

[26] Gwee KA, Wee S, Wong ML, et al. The prevalence, symptom characteristics, and impact of irritable bowel syndrome in an Asian urban community. *Am J Gastroenterol* 2004; 99:924-931.

[27] Rajendra S, Alahuddin S. Prevalence of irritable bowel syndrome in a multiethnic Asian population. *Aliment Pharmacol Ther* 2004; 19: 704-706.

[28] Jafri W, Yakoob J, Jafri N, Islam M, Ali QM. Irritable bowel syndrome and health seeking behaviour in different communities of Pakistan. *J Pak Med Assoc* 2007; 57: 285-287.

[29] Jafri W, Yakoob J, Jafri N, Islam M, Ali QM. Frequency of irritable bowel syndrome in college students. *J Ayub Med Coll Abbottabad* 2005; 4: 9-11.

[30] Boivin M. Socioeconomic impact of irritable bowel syndrome in Canada. *Can J Gastroenterol* 2001; 15 (Suppl B): 8B-11B.

[31] Locke III GR, Yawn B, Wollan PC, Melton III LJ, Lydick E, Talley NJ. Incidence of clinical diagnosis of irritable bowel syndrome in a United States population. *Aliment Pharmacol Ther* 2004; 19: 1025-1031.

[32] Rodriguez G, Ruigomez LA, Wallander MA, Johansson S, Olbe L. Detection of colorectal tumor and inflammatory bowel disease during follow-up of patients with initial diagnosis of irritable bowel syndrome. *Scand J Gastroenterol* 2000; 35: 306-311.

[33] Miller V, Whitaker K, Morris JA, Whorwell PJ. Gender and irritable bowel syndrome: in male connection. *J Clin Gastroenterol* 2004; 38: 558-580.

[34] Whitehead WE, Burnett CK, Cook EW,III, Taub E. Impact of irritable bowel syndrome on quality of life. *Dig Dig Sci* 1996; 41: 2248-2253.

[35] Gralnek IM, Hays RD, Kilbourne A, Naliboff B, Mayer EA. The impact of irritable bowel syndrome on health-related quality of life. *Gastroenterology* 2000; 11: 654-660.

[36] Huerta-Icelo I, Hinojosa C, Santa Maria A, Schmulson M. Diferencias en la calidad de vida (CV) entre pacientes con sindrome de Intestino irritable (SII) y la poblacon mexicana evaluadas mediante el SF-36. *Rev Mex Gastroenterol* 2001; 66 (Suppl 2): 145-146.

[37] Schmulson M, Robles G, Kershenobich, Lopez-Ridaura R, Hinojosa C, Durate A. Los pacientes con trastornos funcionales digestivos (TFD) tienen major compromiso de la calidad de vida (CV) evaluadas por el SF-36 comparados con pacientes con hepatitis C y pancreatitis cronica. *Rev Mex Gastroenterol* 2000; 65 (Suppl-Resumenes): 50-51.

[38] Talley NJ, Gabriel SE, Harmsen WS, Zinsmeister AR, Evans RW. Medical costs in community subjects with irritable bowel syndrome. *Gastroenterology* 1995; 109: 1736-1741.

[39] Harvey RF, Salih SY, Read AE. Organic and functional disorders in 2000 gastroenterology outpatients. *Lancet* 1983; 1: 632-634.

[40] American Gastroenterological Association. *The Burden of Gastrointestinal Diseases*. 2001.

[41] Sandler RS, Everhart JE, Donowitz M, Adams E, Cronin K, Goodman C, Gemmen E, Shah S, Avdic A, Rubin R. The burden of selected digestive diseases in the United States. *Gastroenterology* 2002; 122: 1500-1511.

[42] Lea R, Hopkins V, Hastleton J, Houghton LA, Whorwell PJ. Diagnostic criteria for irritable bowel syndrome: utility and applicability in clinical practice. *Digestion* 2004; 70: 210-213.

[43] Gladman LM, Gorard DA. General practitioner and hospital specialist attitudes to functional gastrointestinal disorders. *Aliment Pharmacol Ther* 2003; 17: 651-654.

[44] Thompson WG, Heaton KW, Smyth GT, Smyth C. Irritable bowel syndrome in general practice: Prevalence, characteristics, and referral. *Gut* 2000; 46: 78-82.

[45] Corsetti M, Tack GR. Are symptom-based diagnostic criteria for irritable bowel syndrome useful in clinical practice? *Digestion* 2004; 70: 207-209.

[46] El-Salhy M, Lomholt-Beck B, Hausken T. Chromogranin as a tool in the diagnosis of irritable bowel syndrome. *Scan J Gastroenterol* 2010; 45: 1435-1439.

[47] Pace F, Molteni P, Bollani S, Sarzi-Puttini R, Stockbrügger R, Bianchi Porro G, Drossman DA. Inflammatory bowel disease versus irritable bowel syndrome: a hospital-based, case-control study of disease impact on quality of life. *Scan J Gastroenterol* 2003; 38: 1031-1038.

[48] Spiller R, Aziz Q, Creed F, Emmanuel A, Houghton L, Hungin P, Jones R, Kumor D, Rubin G, Trudgill N, Whorwell P. Guidelines on the irritable bowel syndrome: mechanisms and practical management. *Gut* 2007; 56: 1770-1798.

[49] Sarna SK. Lessons learnt from post-infectious IBS. Front Physiol 2011; 2: 1-13. doi:10.3389/fphys.2011.00049.

[50] Spiller CR. Role of infection in irritable bowel syndrome. *J Gastroenterology* 2007; 42: 41-47.

[51] Spiller R, Garsed K. Postinfectious irritable bowel syndrome. *Gastroenterology* 2009; 136: 1979-1988.

[52] Ghoshal U, Ranjan P. Post-infectious irritable bowel syndrome: the past, the present and the future. *J Gastroenterol Hepatol* 2011; 26 (Suppl 3): 94-101.

[53] Spiller R, Garsed K. Infection, inflammation and the irritable bowel syndrome. *Dig Liver Dis* 2009; 41: 844-840.

[54] Ghoshal UC, Park H, Gwee KA. Bugs and irritable bowel syndrome: the good, the bad and the ugly. *J Gastroenterol Hepatol* 2010; 25:244-251.

[55] Halvorson HA, Schlett CD, Riddle MS. Postinfectious irritable bowel syndrome – a meta-analysis. *Am J Gastroenterol* 2006; 101: 1894-1899.

Index